HOW CORONA TORMENTED MANKIND

The Way Ahead

ALSO, FROM THE SAME AUTHOR

- Management Wisdom of Lord Krishna
- Corporate Mismanagement
- Gandhian Philosophy and Terrorism
- Invincibility of Corruption
- Indo-Pak Relations: Drama or Diplomacy
- Indo-Pak Relations: Beyond Surgical Strike
- Demonetization X-Rayed
- Revenge of Duryodhana
- Indo-Pak Relations: Beyond Pulwama and Balakot
- Dialogue with God

HOW CORONA TORMENTED MANKIND

The Way Ahead

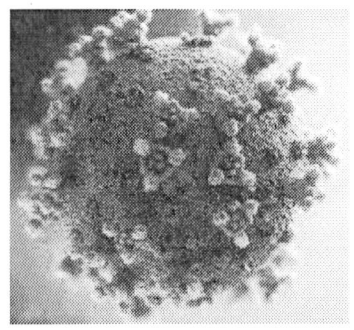

DR U V SINGH

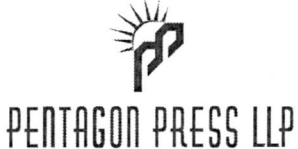

PENTAGON PRESS LLP

How Corona Tormented Mankind

Dr U V Singh

First Published in 2021

Copyright © Reserved

ISBN 978-93-90095-44-5

All rights reserved. No part of this publication may be reproduced, stored in a retrieval system, or transmitted, in any form or by any means, electronic, mechanical, photocopying, recording, or otherwise, without first obtaining written permission of the copyright owner.

Disclaimer: The views and opinions expressed in the book are the individual assertion of the Author. Moreover the Publisher does not take any responsibility for the same in any manner whatsoever. Attributability of the contents lies purely with Author.

Published by
PENTAGON PRESS LLP
206, Peacock Lane, Shahpur Jat
New Delhi-110049
Phones: 011-64706243, 26491568
Telefax: 011-26490600
email: rajan@pentagonpress.in
website: www.pentagonpress.in

Printed at Aegean Offset Printers, Greater Noida, U.P.

*This book is dedicated to my grandchildren:
Aditya Vir Singh, James Leonardo Ripa,
Anya Ripa and Ayaan Vir Singh.*

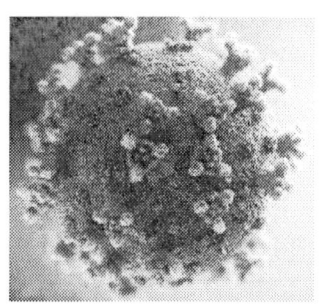

Contents

	Acknowledgements	*xi*
	Introduction	*xiii*
1	Corona's Fast Movement from Wuhan	1
2	Corona Crisis in Italy	4
3	Spain Struggled In and Out of Lockdowns	9
4	France under Coronavirus Attack	12
5	UK's Unimpressive Struggle Against the Pandemic	15
6	Russia under Coronavirus Attack	20
7	Covid-19 Pandemic Changed the World	23
8	Corona Locked Mankind into a Cycle of Infections, Lockouts, Opening-ups, Resurgences and Re-lockouts	27
9	Corona Demolished a Powerful Presidency	30
10	Corona Exposed the Major Faultline of Western Society	33
11	Corona Highlighted Inequality and Poverty in Human Society	36
12	Corona Imposed a Strange Easter and a Joyless Christmas	39

13	Corona Pushed some Governments to Abdicate Governance	41
14	Covid Took a Long Ride on its Victims	47
15	Covid-19 Spawned a Dangerous Digital Divide	49
16	Coronavirus Dived into an International Conspiracy	52
17	Darkest Winter in Human History	55
18	Different Approaches Employed Against Coronavirus	58
19	Europe Struggled to Propel its Stalled Economy	63
20	Some Great Heights of Corona Carnage	67
21	Fulminations of President Trump	71
22	How Should World Change for Safer Future?	76
23	Indian Diaspora and Domestic Migrant Workers	79
24	Indian Lockdown Succumbed to Public Protests	82
25	Lockdowns and Inevitability of Second Wave	85
26	Khaki Brutality in Corona Times	88
27	Lasting Scars of Corona on the Society	90
28	Lifting Lockdowns and Easing of Restrictions	95
29	Long-term Impact of Corona on Human Society	99
30	Many Battles in the Long Corona War	103
31	Master of Resurgence and Lockdown Games	106
32	Medical Fraternity Faced a Situation of No Sure Cure	111
33	Politics of Coronavirus Spread and Containment	113
34	Likely Dark Scenario of the Post-Corona Era	116

35	President Trump Turned into a Super-Spreader of Corona	119
36	Principles Emerging Out of Spread of Corona Pandemic	121
37	Covid-19 Fired a Race for Vaccines Development	125
38	Resurgence: A Basic Strength of Covid-19 Virus	129
39	Revenue Collection Preferred over Public Safety	135
40	Struggle for Lifting Lockdowns	138
41	Suppression of Infection and Mortality Data	141
42	Surge of Corruption in Covid Times	145
43	Conflict Between Saving Lives and Protecting Livelihood	147
44	Truth Became the Greatest Casualty of Covid-19 Pandemic	152
45	Uncertainties Thrown up by the Coronavirus	157
46	Corona: A Fast Unfolding Scenario	160
47	USA Landed In Deadly Grip of Corona	162
48	Massive Efforts towards Vaccines' Development	166
49	India's Disastrous Second Wave	168
50	India's Hidden Covid-19 Deaths	181
51	Certainty of Third Wave in India	183
	Index	185

* * *

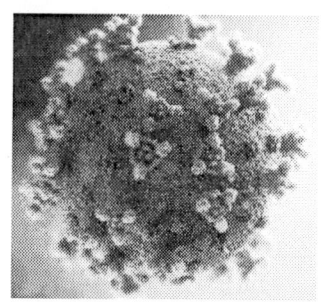

ACKNOWLEDGEMENTS

The lockdown period in India that extended from 24th March 2020 to May end, presented a complex situation related to the extra time at my disposal. As I struggled with the problem, my son-in-law Roberto Ripa suggested that I look at the idea of doing a book on the Covid-19 pandemic that had just started to unfold. When I debated the idea with myself, I found that the pandemic was just a nature's work in progress and figures of infections and deaths in different countries were changing every hour. In view of the complex situation, I too decided to do a running commentary on the dreaded bio-agent and the damage that it caused.

Early in the year, it had put Italy on the mat and aggressively threatened rest of the world to an uncertain fate. In the meantime, my friends at the India Habitat Centre, particularly Arun Kapoor and Raman Chaddha too enquired what I was to engage with during the Covid-19 imposed isolation. They welcomed the idea when I exposed it to them. And afterward, very often, they continued to ask me about the progress in this regard. It was, indeed, difficult to keep track of the unfolding situation imposed by the dreaded pandemic—and without their continued interest in the matter it wouldn't have been possible to persist with the work. I deeply appreciate the active support and feel greatly thankful to all the three well-wishers of mine.

* * *

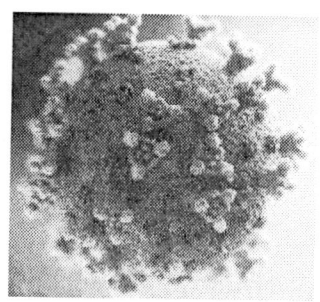

INTRODUCTION

Corona originated in the Wuhan business hub of China in the last quarter of 2019. It's origin, whether from wild animal world or from some virology lab, was clouded in great mystery and caused an international controversy.

> While Americans claimed that the dreaded virus originated from a Chinese virology lab in Wuhan, Chinese authorities protested vigorously. Australia openly towed the American line and some western countries, in a subdued voice, seemed to lay the blame at Chinese doors.

The controversy, or the non-understanding, in this regard continued to simmer all through the year 2020 and 2021. As per nature of the controversy its resolution is decidedly impossible. WHO was seen initially promoting the Chinese line and, as a consequence, earned American displeasure leading to Trump administration suspending financial assistance to the world body. Chinese resisted the idea of an independent inquiry into the origin of the deadly virus which fuelled the suspicion of dragon's complicity in the matter. WHO coined the term 'Covid-19' for the great bio-agent.

> Right in early months of 2020, the Covid-19 pathogen took an air ride with business and pleasure travellers to the west; southern Europe was its first preferred destination to multiply and turn into

> *a deadly pandemic. Italy was first to encounter the vicious attack of the new virus. Spain and France were second to fall prey to the inadequately understood pathogen.*

It didn't take long to extend its grip to UK, Russia, and Germany—and soon, like wildfire, it covered the whole world. The first wave of Covid-19 continued to crush the European continent with varying intensity all through the first three quarters of the year, turning into a more vicious second wave in the fourth quarter when hospital admissions surged and the whole medical infrastructure was overwhelmed as never before. It deprived the EU region, UK, USA, and several other countries of the western world of traditional Christmas/New Year festivities and associated business opportunity to the long-stressed economies.

> *By the second quarter of the year 2020, the deadly virus had covered almost whole the world, including the icy continent.*

Across Atlantic, Brazil and USA turned into preferred battle grounds for massive attack by the great virus. Autocratic and inefficient administrations in both the cases helped the deadly virus to enjoy an unhindered movement and multiplication. While the Brazilian President Jair Bolsonaro called it a **'little flu'**, US President Trump spread several untruths about the deadly virus. Latin American countries, other than Brazil, too didn't perform any better when they were threatened by the great virus. On the other hand, Asian countries except India, Pakistan and Iran, performed better against the deadly pandemic. East Asian countries namely South Korea, Japan, Taiwan, New Zealand, Australia, Vietnam, and Singapore exhibited much better action efficiencies against the pandemic, despite being in proximity of China wherefrom the deadly virus had originated.

> *A study of the movement of the Covid-19 westward suggested that small countries which were ruled by technologically/ financially qualified political personnel or executives who had little or no conflict*

with their medical and scientific advisors, performed better against the dreaded Corona.

African countries, except South Africa, too exhibited better fighting ability against the surging virus, possibly because of their earlier experience of fighting against Ebola and other pandemics. And the Arab world too escaped relatively lightly in its encounter with the dreaded virus.

India's record of its fight against the Corona pandemic seemed initially a mixed one—official circles claiming that it did better than rest of the world while numerous experts thought otherwise. Its record of unplanned lockdown, March through May 2020, was at best controversial as it had pushed millions of industrial/commercial workers from large towns and business/industrial hubs on to roads as their incomes had stopped and they had no resources to survive in urban slums—and, for better or worse, walked to their villages since all transports stood grounded during the lockdown.

Thirsty, hungry, and tired, several of them fell dead on roads, uncared for and unattended by central as well as state governments. The unplanned lockdown had turned into a great human tragedy.

As the year 2020 reached closure the whole world, irrespective of geography, felt greatly tormented as never before in human history.

Over 80 million people were reported infected by the virus during its unrestricted run during the Covid year 2020. The second wave in April/May 2921 was a disaster of unprecedented proportions that put loss of life into several millions. Some sources put the figure several times higher than the officially claimed ones. And in addition to loss of millions of lives the inadequately understood pandemic caused massive social and financial injuries to the innocent public.

In several countries not only medical infrastructures were overwhelmed, in numerous cases burial grounds too fell short while dealing with unexpected demand.

USA, the world's most technologically advanced country, was seen performing most poorly when faced with the pandemic and it had lost over 4,00,000 lives by end of the Covid year. India and Brazil occupied the second and third positions in terms of losses suffered at hands of the Covid-19.

> *The crisis further deteriorated in the first Qtr of 2021 and by the 3rd week of February the US telly of deaths had crossed half a million mark; Brazil crossed half of this figure and Mexico grabbed the third place pushing India to the 4th place with over 3,70,000 officially reported deaths. Actual loss of human life was in fact a minimum 8-10 times higher. And the virus showed no signs of either getting tired or taking some rest.*

In face of the dreaded virus a large number of governments felt confused as how to deal with the Covid challenge. When to lockdown and for how long was seen as a perpetually perplexing question—and opening up of closed economies was equally uncertain and painful. Covid-19 imposed several unpleasant and stressful situations on the mankind, the important ones dealt with in this work were as under:

- The most stressful was people's inability to hold hands of their relatives dying lonely death in hospital ICUs. They weren't allowed inside Covid facilities and patients faced dreadfully lonely departures from the world.
- Staying home in cramped premises with children and elderly during long lockdowns created stressful living environment which eventually, in innumerable cases, led to genesis of depression and also generated conflict between couples and also between seniors and junior members of numerous households.
- On the business front, small businesses such as restaurants and bars suffered the most—innumerable ones collapsed in face of restrictions imposed on sit-down dining and related occupancy aspects.

- Tourism, hospitality, and aviation suffered so much that massive un-employments were created leading into huge social discomforts. A few governments in the developed world offered unemployment allowances while vast majorities in the developing world suffered painful deprivations. Suicides and divorces became common in face of the resultant situation.

- Education of children suffered a great deal, especially those who couldn't afford smart phones and internet were the worst sufferers. A painful divide was created in the student community at all levels. Significant dropouts amongst students from middle and poor sections of the society formed the most unpleasant consequence. Innumerable careers were cut short prematurely or wholly lost tragically.

- *Poverty was seen spiking irrespective of involved societies' state of economic development—not even USA, the world's richest country could escape the situation.*

- GDPs of countries across the whole world suffered slump in range of 10-20 percent. Many governments resorted to launching massive recovery packages.

- Globalisation in conduct of international businesses related to manufacturing as well as flow of services suffered a great deal.

- Relations turned unpleasant between USA and China as the latter's complicity regarding the origin and spread of the Corona virus grew as time passed. Australia lost a significant chunk of its exports to China as the latter reacted to the former actively demanding an independent probe into the matter.

- International organisations, especially the WHO, were seen growing less effective because of the Covid related-19 tensions between some countries.

- President Trump's re-election chances in November 2020

were damaged due to inefficient handling of the Covid situation by his autocratic administration.

- While the medical community world over bravely faced the dreadful challenge thrown up by the unpredictable bio-agent, numerous of these frontline fighters lost their lives in the unequal fight between the mighty nature, on one hand and the stressed humankind, on the other.

- On the other side, there were only a few positives resulting out of the Covid dictated situation. Online conduct of businesses received an unprecedented boost as people were immobilised due to lockdowns and other movement restrictions. Vigorous vaccine development efforts and cooperation by numerous governments and organisations was the other bright side of the Covid dictated situation.

India's gross mismanagement of the second wave of the pandemic in 2nd quarter of 2021 turned most disastrous and the Hindutva stained Modi government lost its credibility (detailed under episode 50 of this work).

These and numerous other related situations that traumatized the mankind form the basic contents of this work.

* * *

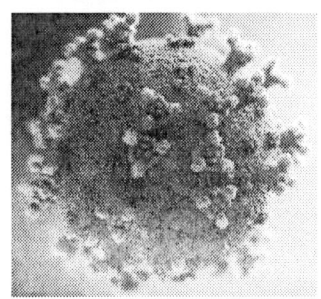

EPISODE 1

CORONA'S FAST MOVEMENT FROM WUHAN

Coronavirus had emerged in the Wuhan city of China, an industrial and business hub, right in November 2019 and it surged December onwards, with break-neck speed, covering the whole world in an unprecedented manner. While China struggled with the disease, the World Health Organization (WHO) gave it a new designation, namely the Covid-19, and right in the first month of the New-Year warned the world about the devastation that it could cause. Initially, China didn't give out adequate information and/or warning about severity of the Pandemic.

> *Some experts felt that China attempted initially to hide the explosion of the deadly virus from the world. While it shut local transport and imposed a strict lockdown, international air travel continued to carry the highly virulent pathogen to numerous state capitals and commercial hubs in the world.*

By end of the first month of the New-Year the Pandemic started raising its ugly head in numerous countries. South Korea, Japan, Malaysia, Singapore, Iran, Pakistan, Italy, and Spain were first to report the infection. They suffered the initial losses of human life that the virus inflicted.

> *Initially, the deadly Pandemic had taken a ride with high flyers and the high healed who travelled by air for business and/or pleasure. It has been claimed that over a million Chinese flew out at the time of the Chinese New-Year—thus seeding the virus all over the world, more intensively in Europe and North America.*

Bergamo town in Northern Italy was the first great victim of this movement of the infection. Not for long the disease stayed with top of the population pyramid—and with the speed of an avalanche it moved to the second and middle strata of population. In a short period, over four and a half thousand people became its unfortunate victim in the small town.

WHO gave another warning and specified precautions like need for frequent washing of hands and avoiding close contact with those who were infected by the deadly virus. Infection was now seen multiplying at breakneck speed in Italy, Iran, and Spain. Hospital wards filled quickly, and the affected countries counted their dead now in thousands. Shortage of the PPE kits for the care giving staff—and ventilators for the critically ill patients became items of great urgency. These critical items were imported by many countries but very few had stocks to spare—or had capacity to manufacture large quantities in short time. By middle of March 2020, the dreaded disease had spread to over 150 countries. Disease's spread and death rates by the Easter Sunday had climbed so fast that keeping a track became difficult. Soon USA left Italy and Spain behind in relation to number of deaths and infections—total number of infections confirmed through tests crossed 15,00,000 and deaths too had crossed the 1,00,000 mark by end of May 2020.

> *President Trump and WHO ran into a spate, blaming each other for not having done enough—and the deadly virus moved unhindered on its massive killing spry.*

President Trump's criticism of WHO, as well as that of China had become sharp by end of April 2020. It was claimed that WHO sided with China in regard to the latter's failure to contain the virus right to Wuhan. USA also suspended its financial contribution to WHO and talked of investigations into the matter. Australian Prime Minister, Scott Morrison, too was seen making remarks critical of China's role in the spread of the deadly virus to all over the world. European countries that suffered a lot at hands of the virus, however, stayed calm in this regard. Silently, they were however supporting the President Trump's contention in this regard.

The deadly virus continued to intensify in South American and African countries. Not only it killed people in hundreds of thousand, economies of most of the countries infected by the dreaded pandemic were crippled beyond repair in the short term. The deadly march of the virus continued unhindered all through the year 2020 and the controversy of its origin and spread too lingered on unabatedly.

* * *

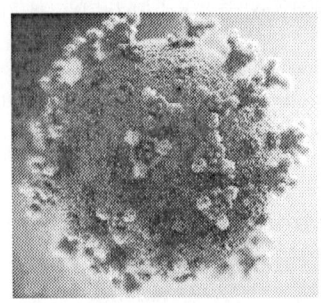

EPISODE 2

CORONA CRISIS IN ITALY

Italy had substantial trade and tourism connections with China. A major part of its iconic brands and goods were manufactured in China. And Italy also imported a large quantity of cheap Chinese goods for sales locally as well as for supplying the same to neighbouring countries (particularly its own brands custom manufactured). This necessitated substantial movement of people, the traders, and salesmen, to and from China. Italy's northern city Milano, a well-known fashion, tourism, and commercial centre, is the prime air travel hub of the country. It is in the Northern Province called Lombardy. In the month of January 2020, the devil of Corona rode to Italy with business travellers and tourists from the east. Some experts were of the view that Corona infection initially had moved to Italy from Germany.

> *China, while it strictly locked down Wuhan (where the deadly Coronavirus originated) and suspended all local transports, had kept the to-and-fro air travel going on in full swing. It even protested when some countries restricted or stopped flights to Wuhan.*

China didn't want the world to form an adverse impression that could adversely affect its international trade. Thus, knowingly, or unknowingly, it promoted spread of the Corona almost world over. And it seemed that the countries which had more frequent and intense trade and travel connections with China were the first ones to see emergence of Corona infection in their local populations. South Korea, Japan, Taiwan, Malaysia, Singapore, Iran, Pakistan, Italy, and Spain were thus gifted with the deadly pandemic in the first phase of its movement out of Wuhan.

> *China in the initial stage of Wuhan pandemic's explosion didn't inform the world about the seriousness of the matter while locally it acted at breakneck speed—testing, tracing isolating, and treating those found infected with the deadly virus. It was the WHO that belatedly warned the world about the seriousness of the matter— and many countries including India, Brazil, UK, and USA didn't take the matter with needed seriousness.*

Italy was somewhat slow to react to the unfolding threat of the pandemic. It was unduly late in closing schools, malls, markets, restaurants, and bars etc and the deadly virus had a free field day. Similarly, its testing, identification and isolation actions were slow to unfold. Free movement of people who brought in the infection to the country resulted into their carelessly mingling with local population. Visits by such infection carriers to old-age homes to meet their relations compounded the situation. As per some experts, the warm Italian culture wherein people loved to greet each other by cheeky contacts possibly contributed to the fast spread of the virus in the society. By middle of March 2020, its graph of infections was rising straight up and daily deaths reached into hundreds.

> *Soon, Italy's medical system, especially in Bergamo town, was seen cracking down under the unexpected flood of sick and infected. Hospital beds fell short of demand and there were not enough ICU beds to accommodate the critically ill. And hospitals ran into shortage of PPEs and the medical staff was seen compromising through the usage of laundry bags for protection. And there were not enough ventilators for the critically sick. Medical staff*

> *highlighted the shortage of essentials and were worried about their own safety and feared that they could carry infection home and infect their own nears and dears.*

Doctors and nurses started falling prey to the deadly disease and the Italian authorities, left imbalanced, made request to USA for its military personnel stationed there to assist in handling the situation. By end of March 2020, the beleaguered nation's death count reached over 10,000, the highest in the world at that time.

Now its famous city squares in Milano and Rome looked dreadfully deserted. The famous St. Peters' Square in Rome was so dreadfully deserted that even Pope was seen rendering his customary sermon to the empty space. Milan's city square which normally teamed with tourists rubbing each other too had a similar fate.

> *By end of the first week of April 2020, its death toll had crossed 17,000. Army trucks were called in to carry and shift the dead to storage and/or burial grounds. Most of the churches were closed and many amongst the dead had to forgo the normal funeral services.*

Italy made furious requests for international help but nothing substantial came its way. The Italian Prime Minister demanded that EU administration come up with a large rescue package (which materialised only in July after bitter and stressful negotiations) to help the severely suffering countries of the South, including itself and Spain, to help them recover from the deadly setback. Brussels was, however, reluctant as some countries especially the Netherlands, Denmark, Austria, and some others were not receptive to the idea. Germany had pushed the idea vigorously and finally a 750 billion Euro rescue package (390 billion as non-returnable and rest as credit) was approved after the 4th meeting of leaders, only the last being an in-person one.

> *By end of April 2020, Italy had suffered around 30,000 deaths at hands of the dreaded Covid-19 and economy of the country was severely dented.*

With the stabilisation of the infection and flattening of the fatalities' curve, the greatly battered country now wrestled with the intricacies of lifting the lockdown and opening-up of the economy. Initially, it allowed small shops and selected businesses to open with conditions of maintaining social distancing etc. Keeping in view the need for some exercise and fresh air for the people, it went ahead to allow them small walks and cycling etc but opening-up its garden and parks had to wait till the second week of May 2020. Schools continued to remain closed as a safety measure. With a lot of caution and hesitations other businesses too started opening-up and commenced working with distancing and occupancy restrictions.

Some commentators assessing the crippling damage suffered by Italy's already shaky economy had stressed the danger of *'New Poverty'* taking hold of the situation. Also, it was feared that in South of the country, dreaded Mafia elements might take advantage of the situation and regain ground there. Fortunately, nothing like this happened.

All through the second and third weeks of May 2020, Italy continued to struggle with necessity of gradual and controlled opening-up measures. Danger of resurgence of the pandemic and the need for public safety was its prime concern.

Finally, in the first week of June 2020, not only the hugely stressed economy was fully opened up, but tourism also related activities were allowed as a priority area. As a connected move, Italy allowed all European tourists to come and enjoy its iconic tourist places and beaches during rest of the summer.

But the fear of resurgence continued to dog the greatly stressed nation as several countries like Spain, France, UK, and Germany, amongst others, suffered the second wave of Corona infections July through end August. And as a result, it could draw only very limited advantage of the 2020 summer tourist season. Schools opened in early September, but the economy continued to struggle a great deal.

> *Italy's relief from the dreaded Corona was not to last for long as resurgence is the most sustained and inviolable nature of this virus.*

And when the whole Europe was downed by a second wave of the pandemic in October, it had to reluctantly re-impose restrictions on movement of people and working of businesses. Central region of the country had now turned into a hotspot and it was feared that the second wave could be more destructive than the first one. Hence, restrictions were tightened, and face masks were made compulsory for those who moved out of their homes. Schools, however, stayed open but many office goers worked from home.

> *People weren't happy facing restrictions. Corona fatigue was seen taking over a section of the population. A large number of people vigorously protested in Milano, Turin and several other business and tourism centres.*

Availability of some effective vaccines by the year end or early 2021 was now the only light visible beyond the dreadful pandemic tunnel. The festive season of Christmas and New Year remained hugely subdued since, like rest of the EU, Italy too was re-crushed by a vicious second wave of the dreadful virus.

* * *

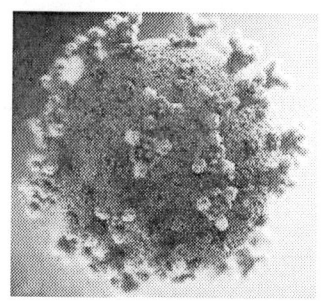

EPISODE 3

SPAIN STRUGGLED IN AND OUT OF LOCKDOWNS

On a Tuesday, after a sombre Easter—and after having suffered several weeks' long drubbings at hands of Coronavirus, Spain decided to partially ease the lockdown. It had suffered the 2nd heaviest death toll (after Italy) in the whole European Union.

> Spain is a tourism dependent and services-based economy. Madrid and Barcelona, both are amongst the most popular tourism hubs in the continent.

Spain's bull fighting festivities and tomato-fight rituals are famous all around the world. Its football clubs too are legendry where matches attract huge gatherings. Millions of visitors from all over the world land here every year—and the end of 2019 and the first quarter of 2020 weren't an exception in any manner.

Covid-19 infection rode to Spain with the flood of air travellers (a) directly from China, on one hand and (b) the already infected Europeans and Americans who landed there for the year-end and New-Year festivities, on the other. Very much like Italy and France, Spain didn't take the threat of the deadly Corona ingress seriously. Incoming dollars and an environment of festivities had blinded sensitivities of the merry-making nation. By end of February 2020, its hospitals started filling up with sick and dying. All through March 2020, Spain suffered heavy casualties at hands of the dreaded disease. Week after week, its daily death counts of the Corona victims competed with those of Italy, far ahead of similar toll in case of France and UK at that time.

> *Early into the first week of April 2020, Spain exceeded a death toll of 13,000 Corona victims. By now its medical services were in total disarray; there was no space left in hospitals wherein even corridors were full of sick and dying.*

They ran short of PPEs and masks for the care giving staff—and there was a terrible shortage of ventilators, the use of which was rationed depending upon the survival chances of patients. Field hospitals were raised in a hurry and morgues ran out of space to store the dead. In order to tide over the situation some ice rings were taken over to store the dead.

Since churches didn't operate for funeral services, the dead suffered consequences of losing funeral rituals and prayers. A large percent of doctors and nurses caught the infection and several of them died in the process. The whole society ran out of options and appealed for international assistance. Italy and Spain together approached the European Union for a large financial assistance package which came through only when Italy hinted at possibility of the EU losing its very existence as an economic grouping of nations.

On Tuesday i.e., the 14th of April 2020, when Spain allowed limited economic activity by partially lifting the lockout, it risked the danger of eventual re-surge. The second surge luckily did not materialise as opening up was gradual and well monitored. Initially only such businesses were opened where social distancing was feasible. Parks, restaurants, and schools opened with restrictions. In Madrid and Barcelona, the two large urban hubs of business and hospitality, residents who for weeks were locked up in most inconvenient settings saw relief of movement and fresh air after middle of May 2020. Death toll by this time at hands of the deadly pandemic had crossed 28,000 and the tourism and services based Spanish economy was gasping for survival.

> *Around 70-80 percent of these victims of the Coronavirus pandemic in the country were senior citizens, mostly living in care homes and it is said that a whole generation was lost. In order to remember them and their contributions to the Spanish society a 10 day long national mourning was declared in the country. For the purpose national flag was lowered and prayers were held in churches.*

Reacting to the situation, opening up of businesses and industry was speeded up and the greatly stressed country expressed a desire to welcome tourists during the fast-approaching summer season. But the great eagerness exhibited by Spain to encash its expected summer tourist influx was not to the taste of the vengeful virus. It surged in bars, restaurants, malls and on beaches to the extent that in the 2nd half of September Madrid and several other parts of the country had to suffer a second lockdown. It seemed that Corona didn't like any unnecessary hurry. And all through the last quarter of the pandemic year Spain, like rest of the Europe, continued to suffer at hands of the deadly virus. It became part of the notorious second wave of Europe that extended well into the New Year.

* * *

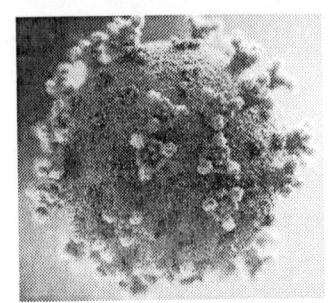

EPISODE 4

FRANCE UNDER CORONAVIRUS ATTACK

During a press conference, President Macron at end of the 3rd week of April 2020 admitted that the country wasn't ready to effectively counter the Coronavirus pandemic. In fact, the threat of the pandemic that had exposed its deadly fangs in Wuhan, a business and industrial hub in China, in December 2019—and then its severe outburst near home in Italy, wasn't taken with needed seriousness by the French establishment.

> *To and fro air traffic and other travel tourism related movement had infused a heavy load of Corona infection into the high fashion and hospitality practicing French society.*

All through the first two months of the New Year and right into the month of March 2020, virus load continued its inflow. There was an obvious lack of coordination between the politics and science in the country. French President's approval ratings were now coming down and he was not progressing towards assuming the EU's leadership that he had dreamt for long. Consequently, the situation of uncertainty and unduly delayed decision on lockdown to curtail movement and mixing up of people had worsened the situation.

Country's medical infrastructure hadn't readied itself with needed beds, ICUs and ventilators etc. during the early months of the year. And there weren't enough PPEs too available for protecting the frontline workers i.e., doctors and nurses to effectively manage a crowded rush of Corona patients. Country's numerous old age-care homes were hopelessly unprepared for facing a serious challenge from the great pandemic moving in unhindered.

> *Confused and disoriented, Macron government salvaged the situation to some extent by imposing a strict lockdown on 17 March 2020, when the Corona patients' death toll was tending to equal that of its neighbours, namely Italy and Spain. Only bakeries, pharmacies, meat retailers and some other essential services were allowed to remain open and functioning.*

Deserted iconic streets, museums and churches in key French cities missed Easter festivities as a surprising and painful event. By end of April 2020, French economy had suffered an incalculable setback; its GDP was estimated to have retreated by 8-10 percentage points—and by the same measure President Macron's reputation as a performing leader was dented equally severely.

The situation in the country was so bad that its iconic aircraft career Charles De-Gaulle too was incapacitated on account of infection of its crew members by the dreaded virus—and had to be docked for curative measures.

By end of the first week of May 2020, death toll in the country had crossed 25,000 and its elders' care homes were devastated.

> *Celebrations for the 75th anniversary of the of the WWII Victory day were dreadfully subdued. There was not a soul on the iconic avenues and squares of Paris—and President Macron had to offer tributes to unknown soldiers near the 'Arc de Triumph' on the historic occasion in total isolation.*

All through the month of May 2020, France, like other Corona victimised countries, struggled to gradually attempt with opening-up the lock-downed and severely crippled economy.

The June/July efforts of the country to salvage summer tourist season in order to allow some breathing space to the country's vast hospitality sector was punished by the non-forgiving virus with a massive resurgence in the month of August. A re-lockdown was the only unavoidable choice for the Corona tormented nation. Situation worsened in September when in middle of the month, daily count of reported infections touched the peak of 30,000. Resultantly, hospitals got crowded with infected people seeking treatment and, as an associated consequence, daily deaths figures crossed the level of 200 a day. Panicked by the hopeless situation 11 large urban centres in the country, including its capital, were put under strict night curfew. Restaurants and bars were ordered to close sharp at 10 PM in order to curtail human interaction. People protested for lost freedom but there was no choice to the hugely stressed society. Situation continued to deteriorate and towards end of October, French government was forced to impose strict national lockdown for a month and people protested vehemently. The situation didn't improve in November and it seemed certain that the country was headed towards facing a very sombre Christmas/New Year holiday season. It became a part of the notorious second wave of Europe that extended well into the year 2021.

* * *

EPISODE 5

UK'S UNIMPRESSIVE STRUGGLE AGAINST THE PANDEMIC

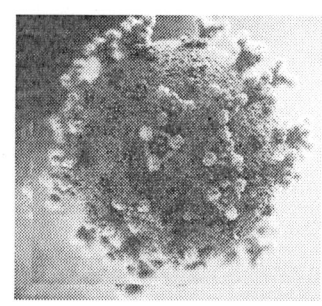

United Kingdom too, like several other European states, was slow and indecisive in realising gravity of the threat of the deadly Covid-19 virus. It didn't close air travel even when Italy, Spain and France suffered huge number of infections and deaths at hands of the invisible enemy. Also visible was the mismatch of political and scientific opinions, utterances, and actions in this regard.

> *The lockdown decision was significantly delayed letting the dreaded virus to have a stormy run all over the country. The country was slow in organising testing, contact tracing, identification, and isolation of the infected. First, Prince Charles fell sick on account of Corona infection—and then at end of March 2020, Mr. Boris Johnson, the country's Prime Minister, too was down with the dreaded disease. He was rendered non-functional for several weeks in March and April, spending almost two weeks at the St. Thomas Hospital, including three days in ICU. And when out of the hospital, he spent weeks at Chequers, the Prime Minister's country house, to recover and recuperate. This episode too possibly somewhat hampered the battle of the beleaguered kingdom in its struggle against the surging enemy.*

On 27th April, Boris Johnson was back in the office and during his first post-Corona press conference said that the lockdown was to be continued. He stressed that any hurried decision regarding opening up the economy ran risk of a second wave of infection which could be even more dangerous to the British society and its economy than the first one. Caution and patience were advocated as the official line of action.

From mid-March through whole April, the medical infrastructure of the country, known as NHS, was seen cracking at its seams under pressure of inflow of the Corona inflected people. There was shortage of hospital beds, ICUs, and ventilators for critically ill patients. Shortage of PPEs, including face masks and gloves for doctors and nurses attending to patients threatened to infect and incapacitate several of them.

> *Over a 100 of these frontline medical warriors had fallen victim to the deadly Covid-19 by this time. During the period, long lines of ambulances were seen outside several hospitals of the country. And over 20,000 people had fallen to the dreaded attack of the great Covid-19 invasion during his period.*

Several days delay in arrival of a plane load of PPEs from Turkey at a weekend in the third week of April 2020, wasn't less than sort of a drama dictated by outside dependence of the country for simple but critical tools needed in the epic battle against the dreaded disease. Medical staff, the frontline warriors, had to resort to **'Jugad'** in order to ensure some protection in the dreaded battle.

Situation at the country's resources-starved old-age homes was even more desperate than what was encountered by the NHS facilities. Retired doctors and nurses had to be recalled for facing the dreadful situation. By end of April 2020, the fight against the dreaded virus had claimed several lives of these senior frontline workers.

> *The medical professionals paid dearly for the negligence and indecisiveness of the government in the initial period of the deadly Corona's invasion.*
>
> *Several scientists, medical experts and intellectuals questioned the government's decisions and non-decisions and their timings in regard to the country's not very efficient struggle against the dreaded disease.*

Dictated by the grim situation resulting out of the Covid-19 invasion Queen's 94th birthday celebrations which included a traditional gun salute, had to be cancelled.

Towards end of April 2020, the British government was seen contemplating opening-up of business activities which were crippled during the lockdown. In the meantime, efforts to develop a vaccine against the Coronavirus were intensified and the Oxford University's scientists reported significant progress in this regard. The fight against the dreaded disease continued into May and June 2020, as it was not an isolated battle but a long-drawn dreaded war with a lots of ups and downs.

By end of the first week of May, UK had overtaken Italy in terms of deaths at hands of the Covid-19 pandemic. In terms of the loss of human lives suffered at hands of the pandemic, UK was now second in the world, just behind only the United States of America.

UK's grim battle against the Corona pandemic continued unabated all through June, July, and August 2020. The need to open businesses and industry in order to allow some respite to the economy continued to weigh heavily on the government. In the meantime, the summer rush of holiday makers to and from the country added to complications, pressing it for decisions on quarantining the people returning from holidays. Several other countries in Europe too had imposed quarantine restrictions on UK travellers. And in the meantime, the virus continued to surge and resurge wherever authorities made mistakes in terms of imposing needed restrictions on group entertainment and working in congested spaces. Several factories processing meat were seen suffering deadly resurgences.

> *Growing unemployment, homelessness and economy walking into depression had complicated job of the government—and the unequal struggle was now seen moving into the last quarter of the year 2020. In middle of October 2020, several areas in UK saw dangerous level of resurgence of the pandemic—and the government announced imposing three tier of restrictions on working of already crippled businesses and interaction of people.*

In early October 2020, the dreaded virus was seen going out of control as daily deaths resulting out of the same had crossed the figure of 200—and it threatened to accelerate out of control. The so-cornered government debated the situation and despite difference of opinions it decided against imposing countrywide lockdown in order to meet the situation. The Prime Minister said that the country was at a precarious tipping point and without restrictions the second wave bashing the British society could inflict serious loss of life and businesses. Hence, he advised people to work from home, close eating places and bars etc at 10 PM, and observe all the suggested measures related to face-masking, social distancing, and social mixing in order to enable the nation to avoid suffering huge costs.

Several other countries in Europe, including Spain, France, Netherlands, Austria, and Germany, amongst others, suffered devastating second wave of virus surging almost unrestrictedly. And UK, reacting to the situation, finally imposed three tier restrictions on people and businesses in order to deal with the surging pandemic. In the second week of December, UK government not only approved the Pfizer vaccine for emergency usage but went in for a campaign to vaccinate its frontline workers in hospitals and the more vulnerable people in age-care homes. The struggle against the Covid-19 moved into the year 2021 after substantially dampening the Christmas/New Year festivities.

> *Subsequently, a strain of the virus called UK variant hugely complicated recovery efforts of the greatly stressed kingdom. And it quickly travelled to India to create a truly disastrous second wave of the pandemic killing millions of people and maiming several times more through the so called 'Long Covid.'*

* * *

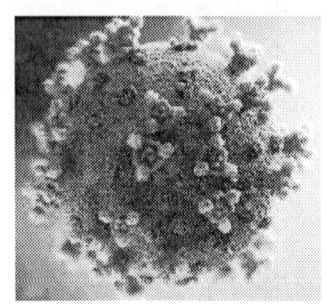

EPISODE 6

RUSSIA UNDER CORONAVIRUS ATTACK

Russia had substantial exposure to and fro business and non-business contacts with China. It was relatively slow to assess the seriousness of the Coronavirus blow-up in Wuhan, a business hub in China—and its possibility of soon reaching across the border to Russia.

> *Falling crude oil prices had not only engaged Russian authorities' attention a great deal but had left it worried and this possibly was the reason why Wuhan episode did not set it into preparations to face the advancing threat of the deadly virus. After knocking Italy and Spain to ground, the deadly pandemic walked into Russia with an unabated ferocity.*

By end of the second week of April 2020, Russian hospitals had started to fill with Corona infected patients—and despite having been put under strict lockout, Moscow had turned into a pandemic's hotspot—and towards middle of the 3rd week of April, President Putin looked worried during press briefings on the subject. He indicated that within a few days hospitals in the Russian capital might run out of beds on account of the flood of Covid-19 patients.

> *Outside one Corona specific hospital located on outskirts of Moscow, miles long queues of ambulances were seen waiting to off-load the patients that they had brought in for admission.*

President Putin had never faced such a serious threat to the nation in the past 20 years for which he has been in power. It is said that even Chernobyl nuclear meltdown had not posed such a serious threat in terms of danger to human life and to the Russian economy.

When on 28th February 2020 Italy requested for international help towards encountering the Covid-19 catastrophe that had unfolded in the South European state, Russia had sent a group of over 30 doctors and paramedics to help in the dire situation. Italy had encountered the deadliest face of an invisible enemy. Hence, it can't be presumed that Russia was not aware of what the deadly disease could do to the population and the medical infrastructure of an affected country. It had also seen its neighbouring Germany to have effectively faced the situation through speedy testing and needed subsequent contact tracings and detention measures. But despite adequate information and some direct experience with the deadly disease its preparations and readiness weren't of a superior level. Possibly, Russia couldn't stir-up the right mix of politics and science well in time necessary for facing the deadly enemy successfully.

Now the otherwise impressive streets of Moscow looked deserted and its massive churches had no human presence.

In the first week of May 2020, cases of Covid-19 infections grew exponentially. Daily escalation in such cases had grown to over 10,000 making the situation truly grim. And supply of PPEs and other protective tools for doctors and nurses had not improved as there was global scramble for the same. In over 200 countries of the six continents now suffering from the great pandemic, every country was looking to procure these essentials for the front-line workers in hospital facilities, large or small. It was reported that several medical workers in Russia contacted the deadly virus and several of them fell prey to the same. Protests of the Russian paramedics and doctors against the dreaded situation brought ridicule and even punishment.

> *Towards end of the first week of May 2020, some front-line medical workers were reported to have fallen from hospital windows and/or balconies. It was feared that the same might not have been result of innocent accident or carelessness on part of the victims.*

During the 2nd and 3rd weeks of May 2020, the pandemic tightened its stronghold on Russia. For over a week in succession, the daily rise of fresh cases of infections spurted by over 10,000. And the total of Russian infections now was only second to that of the USA. It seemed vulnerable and uncertain as how to deal with the pandemic's challenge. For the first time since 1989 when the Soviet empire collapsed and disintegrated, Russia had never been seen in such a helpless state. Shortage of PPEs and other medical essentials for an effective fight against the pandemic persisted and it seemed to adversely affect the morale of the medical community that struggled against the dreaded pandemic on frontlines.

And as a result, President Putin looked worried and uncertain. For the President's own safety from the Covid-19, the worried Russian authorities installed a sanitization tunnel at his official residence and all visitors had to pass through it while being sprayed with sanitizers. By middle of June 2020, Brazil had pushed Russia down to third place in terms of infected people reported.

> *Russia again came under a massive attack of the dreaded virus in October and November 2020 when rest of Europe too faced the destructive second wave of the pandemic. Its hospitals were again overwhelmed under the load of Covid-19 infected patients.*

The hugely stressed nation in the first week of December 2020 hurried up to launch its indigenous vaccine 'Sputnik-V' as a tool to deal with the pandemic's challenge. A massive vaccination program was launched to immunise front-line workers and teachers who had faced the highest exposure. The pandemic greatly dulled Christmas/New Year festivities and marched into the New Year with uncommon defiance. Rest of Europe was in the same boat.

EPISODE 7

COVID-19 PANDEMIC CHANGED THE WORLD

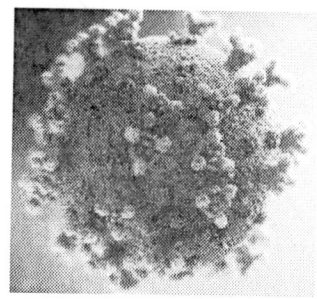

By early April 2020, medical experts, economists, and sociologists in major parts of the world had started to talk and assert that the Covid-19 pandemic was changing the world and the human society so much that almost in all aspects of life, commercial and/or non-commercial, there shall emerge new normal in a wholly unexpected manner.

> *It was stressed that Covid-19 was just a work in progress and that new normal positions shall be created in coming months and years in a manner that no aspect of human life shall be left untouched or in the pre-pandemic state.*

Medical science and its practitioners were challenged immensely by the Covid-19 pandemic; they were no more fully confident of the powers of this field of science against the vicious bio-agent. And while dealing with patients in OPDs, or in their personal chambers, images of medical personnel clad with PPEs, gloves, face masks and sanitizers became increasingly visible. It turned into a new normal in the long-lasting pandemic period.

> *World economy or say economies of all affected nations were mauled significantly. Some components of the economy like aviation,*

> *tourism and hospitality suffered all through the year 2020 and may take years to recuperate and return to the pre-Covid-19 levels. Under-capacity operations, persisting unemployment and financial losses shall be the new normal of this section of the economic environment.*

The concept and practices of the pre-Covid-19 global operations, especially those related to economy stood wholly altered, or significantly challenged. Greater tendency towards self-reliance amongst several nations regarding critical items related to health care became increasingly visible. Custom manufacturing, trade, and related international travel, especially air travel, to supervise and/or speed up such activities became significantly subdued. Online communications in such matters became a rule. Digital turned into a new normal and, indeed, king of most human interactions.

All aspects of the hospitality industry—hotels, restaurants, spas, casinos, and other related components of the entertainment industry, including occupation of beaches and swimming pools either remained closed for long or operated intermittently and on under-capacity. And whenever these activities attempted to open or restart, they quickly led to infection spikes leading to re-closures and/or restrictive working. Manufacturing industry, consumer goods or engineering products, seemed destined to take years to come to pre-Covid-19 levels—and activities related to distribution and retailing of the same continued to lag behind for a long time, often creating frustrations and distress amongst those involved. In several cases of small businesses straightway closures became more convenient than continuing painfully. Operations of malls and large markets continued lingering on an unsustainably thinner level, often threatening closures. GDP expressions of almost all economies of major and minor countries stayed in negative or sub-normal range and improvements were difficult to predict in the troublesome post-Covid-19 environment.

Migrant workers' movement, technical as well as manual,

domestically and/or across borders, remained slow except in case of those desperate for survival.

Several universities and other teaching and training institutions continued to suffer vacancies and under occupations. Career selections and job preferences by fresh graduates suffered a metamorphosis in light of an altered demand scenario. Methods of teaching and intellectual interactions went digital to a very large extent—and those who couldn't afford smart phones or laptops and weren't served well with internet, suffered silently, thus accelerating the gap between haves and have-nots. Some bright students, especially in developing countries, who couldn't face the situation, simply committed suicide.

> *In general, disparity, inequality and poverty showed tends that were uncomfortable and the resultant ugly situation accelerated unabatedly all through the Covid-19 year 2020 and beyond.*

Religious gatherings—churches, mosques, temples, and services rendered therein, were substantially curtailed waiting for normalcy to return. Services related to marriages, deaths, burials, and funerals were allowed much smaller attendance.

Conferences, meetings and even training sessions went virtual on account of compulsions dictated by the Covid-19 pandemic. Classrooms were redesigned to allow larger spacing. Distance education was seen becoming a new normal, though not necessarily more efficient. The Corona pandemic generated and/or accelerated numerous other expected or unexpected trends, almost in all aspects of human life.

International co-operation, UN operations and those of its associate organisations turned low key. International lending and LORR owings suffered a great deal. International groupings such as G-20, G-7 and OPEC etc tended to turn less effective. President Trump's assertions that the Chinese authorities had deliberately misguided the world about Covid-19 pandemic's origin and their failure to restrict the virus to Wuhan itself continued to cause substantial tensions. WHO failed to clear doubts about origin of the virus and its spread which caused differences between US and China to turn sharp, almost into a tsunami of a type of hate virus.

Games arenas, fields and pitches saw much reduced attendance by spectators and fans. Even organisation and operation of Olympic games weren't expected to reach previous levels of celebrations and opulence for years to come.

Arts, artists, galleries, and museums saw much less foot-falls—and with the subdued tourism, wildlife management and protection activities suffered a great deal. In several cases even wildlife viewing turned digital, an astonishing new normal.

> *Covid-19 pandemic continued being a work in progress all through the year 2020 and 2021—and it might take years of concerted efforts and some good vaccines to free the world from the curse of the deadly Corona. And it is assessed that by that time the world, how it worked and interacted, shall stand greatly altered. There shall be many expected and unexpected new normal for the seriously mauled mankind.*

Covid-19 also altered how different societies celebrated festivals and moved around in holiday season. Diwali, the great Indian festival of lights was seen a lot subdued in the active Covid period of November 2020.

In several counties people as well as their governments exhibited signs of having developed active fatigue against normal measures taken to curb the pandemic. Also, the medical community in several countries exhibited active signs of developing fatigue against the dreaded disease. In several European and American counties people protested against Covid related restrictions. And a clear trend was seen emerging in some countries towards a preference to save livelihood against just saving lives. The above and several similar developments more than confirmed that the great Corona had changed the human society to a substantial extent.

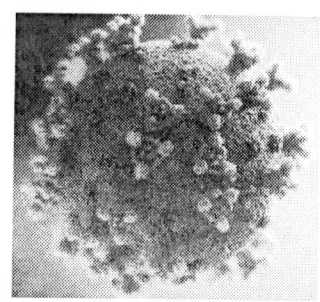

EPISODE 8

CORONA LOCKED MANKIND INTO A CYCLE OF INFECTIONS, LOCKOUTS, OPENING-UPS, RESURGENCES AND RE-LOCKOUTS

> *The tiny virus demonstrated beyond doubt that it was a lot more powerful than the mighty mankind that had made huge strides in various fields of science and technology—and was knocking at the doors of Mars located months of space travel away from the earth.*

The invisible bio-agent's powers were indeed amazing. Emerging in Wuhan town of China in December 2019, it had conquered almost whole the world within 2-3 months. Its speed and swath had pushed the world into confusion as how to deal with the highly deceptive enemy.

First, it pushed Southern Europe to ground and made the countries there to cry for help. Soon, it had gripped UK and USA by neck and strolled with ease of a professional striker into rest of Europe, Americas, Asia, and Africa. Governments all over the world were confused; they didn't know what to do, except pushing deeply scared citizens behind doors through movement restrictions. Thus, commenced the hugely painful cycle of lockdowns, opening-ups, resurgences, and re-lockdowns, briefly code-named here as LORR.

Since the highly deceptive bio-agent's energies and tendencies were unknown, human-beings had no known defence against it; there wasn't any known drug that could be tried for relief, if not cure. And authorities, leave aside the people, didn't know how to protect themselves against its wild march; face masks and PPEs weren't easily available in the initial months of the vicious rampage.

> *People suffered a great deal behind closed doors, many without food and medicines. Not being able to meet nears and dears, for weeks together, was most punishing for the locked-up populace.*

Lockdowns were not a sustainable measure since they directly damaged agencies of livelihood, on one hand and caused dangerous mental stress to people detained inside tiny dwellings, on the other. Children and elderly suffered the most. Jobs were lost and economies nose-dived which further confused governments. They rushed to open-up in an unplanned and hasty manner. People, so freed, mingled vigorously, a good faction not using face masks and not maintaining social distancing. In many countries with high population density social distancing was not practically feasible—and the western world's love for bars, restaurants, gyms, travel, beaches, and malls etc came in the way of successfully dealing with the deadly virus.

> *The cunning virus took advantage of human follies and frailties and surged merrily, infecting a large number and knocking down many. Confused authorities with overflowing hospitals, beds and ICUs fully occupied, and having no more space for critically ill, jumped again to lockdowns, some for weeks and on week-ends, and others going for restricting isolated zones, towns and/or localities. The inherent stress and confusion so created wasn't sustainable. Economies further suffered, accelerating job losses, hunger and destitution on a scale not previously known.*

And consequently, opening-up of businesses and trade being the only option, governing authorities fell into the virus-dictated cycle of LORR. Graveyards were filling fast and not knowing what to do, authorities resorted to confusing measures.

> *President Trump in USA and Jair Bolsonaro of Brazil made maximum contribution to the cycle of LORR that crippled the mankind into a non-performing form.*

Some countries suffered second and third waves of infections right in the first half of the year2020 and in countries like USA and Brazil, the deadly pandemic had an unhindered long run. Europe was crushed by a deadly second wave in October/November and in USA several waves merged into uncontrolled run of the dreaded virus.

> *The virus dictated curse of LORR continued all through the year, destroying economies and crippling societies at will. It seemed as if a mighty hunter had gone berserk in a forest filled with helpless animals. Only a flood of good vaccines could possibly offer relief to the badly cornered human society from a deadly strangle-hold of the murderous enemy.*

India came under a serious grip of the pandemic July through October 2020 when millions of people suffered and innumerable deaths occurred in rural India, a large proportion of which was assigned causes other than the virus. India had no option but to resort to a variety of lockouts in view of its population density and nose-diving economy compounding the situation. In November, the National Capital Region (NCR) suffered another deadly (sometimes called as third wave by local authorities) in the aftermath of Diwali festivities that had turned congested markets of Delhi and adjoining towns into massive hot spots for the virus to breed at an astonishing speed. New hospital beds had to be arranged on emergency basis but in view of sagging economy lockdown was avoided.

The distressed human society now desperately waited for arrival of dependable vaccines and, on this count, there were some bright promises towards end of the year 2020 and the same fructified with the New Year.

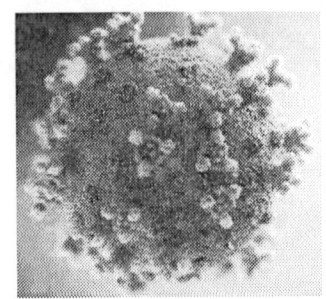

EPISODE 9

CORONA DEMOLISHED A POWERFUL PRESIDENCY

> *Coronavirus was small, rather invisible, yet it didn't shy away from taking on mighty autocrats and often demolished them with professional ease. It pushed them to ground and let them realise that a tiny bio-agent was mightier than them.*

Autocrats and/or dictators in Russia, Brazil, USA, Iran, Turkey, Philippines and arrogant democrats in India and some other countries received the worst drubbings at hands of the Covid-19. South Europeans were crushed simply because they gave an early air ride to the virus from Wuhan. Brazil's autocratic President Jair Bolsonaro called it a *'little flu'* and paid for the folly very dearly. At least in private, he regretted a great deal his belittling comments and learnt to, never in future, underestimate even a tiny enemy. The Chinese dictator, Xi Jinping who lovingly dispatched the great virus to all large business and tourism hubs of the world through air travel comfort was rewarded for, handsomely and respectfully by the mighty pathogen.

> *Most significantly USA, the mightiest nation on earth that happened being governed by an autocratic President, was the preferred choice for the longest and bloodiest drubbing at hands of the tiny virus.*

President Trump had ignored experts' advice in January as well as February 2020 and in March he was busy with his India tour, learning to do *'namaste'* and being photographed in front of the Taj, the world-renowned monument at Agra.

Subsequently, right up to his electoral defeat in November 2020, he made numerous mistakes in dealing with the mighty virus, the prominent of which were:

- He not only disagreed with but even insulted his scientific advisors. One Dr R. Bright, an expert on vaccine development was fired from his job. Aggrieved a great deal, he turned into a whistle-blower and subsequently deposed in a Congressional hearing organised by democrats who had a majority in the house.
- Dr Anthony Fauci of Centre for Disease Control (CDC), a renowned US institution related to public health, was rubbed the wrong way at numerous occasions.
- *President Trump suggested that detergents could be injected into human body to get rid of the Covid-19 virus. It was a crazy thought that germinated in President Trump's mind and, as such, couldn't be explained how it happened despite an army of advisors around him?*
- He differed with Governors on implementation of lockdowns in various states of the oldest democracy of the world. Testing and tracing requirements, as well as availability of PPEs and ventilators made available to the medical staff who endangered their lives while taking care of the Covid-19 patients, were other issues fuelling differences with his experts as well as state authorities.
- The President criticized WHO several times for (a) allegedly concealing facts about the pandemic's origin in Wuhan, and (b) for favouring Chinese when international concerns arose in regard to fixing responsibility for the spread of the deadly

disease. He threatened to stop US aid to the international organisation dealing with public health related issues and attempted crippling its functioning.

- In May 2020, he realised the need for lifting lockouts and opening up of the economy despite the fact that the Covid-19 infection was still surging in the country. He went ahead even to incite his party members to agitate for the opening-up of the economy. He threatened state governors on more occasions than necessary, for disagreeing with him.

Slowly, he lost popularity and gave opportunity to his opponents to go aggressive against him. Over months' long agitation that resulted from killing of an African American at hands of the police in last week of May 2020 (and extended over into June and July) in over 150 cities and towns across the country, was greatly mismanaged by the President. Delayed arrest of the accused police personnel and not slapping up of proper charges against them further ruined Trump's reputation. His decision to deploy national guards against the *'Black Lives Matter'* agitators further ruined his administrative reputation, on one hand and pushed the African American community towards democrats, on the other.

His eagerness and push for opening-up of schools when the deadly virus was surging in almost over 40 states wasn't appreciated by majority of parents and education experts.

The above coupled with numerous other follies of Trump's actions and inaction robbed him of a second term of US Presidency when elections took place in November 2020. While he sulked and refused to accept election results, the mighty Corona mocked at him vigorously.

* * *

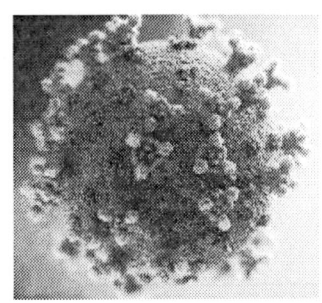

EPISODE 10

CORONA EXPOSED THE MAJOR FAULTLINE OF WESTERN SOCIETY

> *Coronavirus hit hardest the western world which primarily comprises of Europe and Americas, while Asian and African countries (with a few exceptions) escaped lightly.*

In October and November 2020, Corona had almost whole Europe on the mat through what was called the *'second wave'* of the pandemic. Belgium, unable to cope with the vicious attack of the deadly virus, was forced to fly its critical patients to Germany. Italy saw the virus running through its central region in addition to reappearing in the north. In Milano and some other areas people protested vigorously against re-imposition of restrictions on businesses and movement of people. Hospitals were again seen being under stress and, at some places, patients waited for long hours before being taken in. The second wave surpassed the first one in terms of severity as well as spread as daily count of new infections exceeded 40,000. Spain remained under public health emergency for several weeks and here too people protested on loss of freedom to move around and enjoy life.

> *France was one of the hardest hit areas in the continent as at some stages its daily new infections' count had exceeded 60,000, an exceedingly high figure considering its population size and excellent medical facilities.*

UK looked as if its first wave had just metamorphosed into a more vicious second one since there wasn't an apparent gap between the two. It underwent a several weeks long structured lockdown. Towards end of the Covid year 2020 emergence of a new mutant of the virus, popularly called 'British Mutant' greatly complicated the UK's pandemic management scenario. More strict lockdown measures were implemented, and a large number of countries discontinued flights to and from the greatly stressed country. Infections mounted and death toll in UK crossed the unexpectedly high level of 80,000, the highest in the European continent.

Germany too reported daily new cases count of over 20,000 and, next door, Austria suffered a lockdown to get a handle on the growing infections. Even Greece, a country of isolated islands, suffered a serious bout of Covid-19 attack. Russia too suffered a crushing resurge of the virus and since regular medical infrastructure was overwhelmed, field hospitals had to be erected to deal with the situation. In fact, no part of Europe was free of the deadly surge of the virus in the October-December period.

By middle of November, in USA the daily count of new infections had exceeded 1,00,000 and reported hospital admissions crossed the level of 60,000. Presidential election had apparently contributed to the worsening of the situation and defeat of President Trump and his refusal to accept results further complicated the situation.

> *It was perplexing to see how an economically strong and scientifically advanced nation, with highly advanced medical facilities, suffered such a fate.*

By now, it had suffered over 2,40,000 casualties at hands of the great Corona and experts warned that if administration didn't improve it approach hundreds of thousands might further fall prey to the deadly virus before end of the Christmas/New Year period. The experts' apprehension turned true—and by the time Trump was ready to vacate the *'White House'*, daily deaths on account of the furiously surging Corona had crossed the level of 4,000—total of such causalities touching the world's highest level of 4,00,000.

Up north, Canada did a lot better. But down south, the Latin American region's performance in combating the Corona wasn't any better than what was exhibited by the great Superpower to the north.

Why such a poor performance by the western world against a tiny bio-agent, despite its superior technological and economic capabilities, wasn't easily understandable. On considerable analysis, the author came to conclude that the basic fault-line of the western world pertained to its open culture that is characterised by going to pubs/bars, clubs, restaurants, malls, beaches, sports arenas, and museums (just to name a few) that formed necessity for the high human interaction-based travel and tourism dependent economies. It provided a fertile ground to the dreaded virus to breed and quickly jump from person to person in the high human interaction environment. And the democratic nature of governance in most parts of the western world allowed people to ignore administrative instructions a great deal. Additionally, politicians differed with experts that delayed difficult or right decisions needed in challenging situation such as thrown up by a destructive pandemic. This potent mix of the environment and behaviour was loved by the dreaded virus and it did an impressive job in pinning the western world down to the mat, causing massive infections and avoidable loss of life, on one hand and serious damage to numerous economies, on the other.

* * *

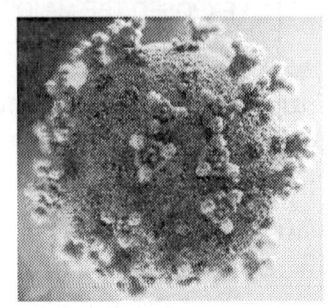

EPISODE 11

CORONA HIGHLIGHTED INEQUALITY AND POVERTY IN HUMAN SOCIETY

Poverty and inequality always existed in the human society. Its form and intensity varied a great deal from country to country and from community to community. The Covid-19 Pandemic exposed its most distressing aspects in a dramatic manner.

> *In USA, the richest nation in the world, registrations of unemployed who wanted relief had climbed to over 40 million (almost a third of the total work force) by end of May 2020. Lines in front of food charities and soup kitchens had lengthened unexpectedly.*

Many people faced difficulty towards paying rent for their small dwellings. Situations were no different in UK, France, Spain, and Italy. In some countries people were seen lowering baskets for help, particularly for food items.

Growing problem of homelessness prompted UK to announce plans to establish 6,000 new homes for those who had nowhere to live. In some South American and African countries things looked desperate.

> *A large population found it difficult to put food on the table and a significant percent of the same could afford only a single meal a day for bare survival.*

Starkest scenes of poverty and inequality became visible in India when, in April and May 2020, hordes of migrant workers who were rendered jobless and homeless in metros and large towns on account of the unplanned lockouts—and were forced to walk long distances to their villages. Homeless, penniless, and hungry, they turned to roads to walk to their homes in states like UP, Bihar, West Bengal, Orissa, MP, and Rajasthan. Road and train transport was unjustifiably denied to them initially for over a month as the Government of India (GOI) and state governments didn't know how to deal with the problem. People walked long distances on foot with small loads, small children, and babies with them. Some families used cycles and rickshaws to move home and several of them were killed on roads by trucks and other vehicles and were left unattended and uncared for. GOI didn't like the scene on roads and instructed police to push the walking masses away from roads—and so foxed, the migrants took to walking on train tracks where several of them were mowed down by goods trains, passenger trains being off the track during the Indian lockdowns.

The size of such crowds moving on roads and rail tracks was estimated being several million strong and the situation was deeply chaotic.

> *Children were dragged sleeping on suite cases and several pregnant women delivered babies on road, rested for an hour or two and then continued their walk home with new-borns in their laps.*

When some trains (called dharmic trains) started in May after a lot of hue and cry, the situation deteriorated a lot further. Illiterate labourers were asked to make bookings online, make several rounds to police and railway stations for confirmation and waited hungry and thirsty for days and weeks. They were charged for travel despite announcement by governments that the travel was paid for by the state. Corruption thrived on misery of poor people.

As if this wasn't enough, trains with migrant workers were sent on longer and/or wrong routes, probably to punish them for bringing a bad name to the publicity conscious Government of India. Some trains roamed aimlessly for days, moving in wrong directions. Passengers weren't provided food and/or water in most cases and there were food and water riots at numerous railway plate-forms. Many people died in trains and on plate-forms unattended for days.

> *The situation was chaotic and the Central Government that ran one of the largest train networks in the world blamed state governments, particularly those run by opposition parties. It was the most unexpected display of inequality and poverty, existence of which in India wasn't a secret and hence it was difficult to understand why such an unwanted display was resorted to by an ideologically intense government that wanted to turn India into a dollar 5 trillion economy, on one hand and make the country a 'Vishwa Guru', on the other.*

The Covid-19 pandemic possibly didn't like existence of extreme poverty and inequality in the human society and hence, it was relentless in exposing the same. It succeeded brilliantly in its drive.

* * *

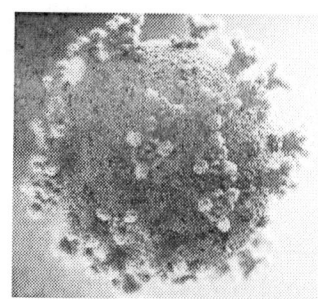

EPISODE 12

CORONA IMPOSED A STRANGE EASTER AND A JOYLESS CHRISTMAS

> 2020 Easter celebrations in the Corona environment represented the strangest situation to the Catholic world. It has been a festival that celebrated new life i.e., the rise of Christ from grave three days after his hoisting on the cross. It is normally marked with massive festivities, interestingly decorated and vibrant churches, sounding of bells and rituals filled prayers.

In 2020, it was marked with deaths and morbidities world over. There was hardly any country in the world, small or big and rich or poor that hadn't registered a large number of uncommon deaths at hands of the deadly Pandemic. World's superpower too was in constrictive grip of an unyielding Corona. It couldn't use any of its weaponry, nuclear or otherwise, to set itself free. Its space-based forces and artificial intelligence (AI) too were clueless as how to respond. Its bureaucracy ran as headless chicken searching for simple necessities like PPE kits, face masks and ventilators.

> At the iconic St Peters Square in Rome, Pope was seen standing just with five or six of his assistants, suitably distanced, to deliver the Easter sermon. It was, indeed, strange. Catholic world had never

> *suffered such a humiliation even in the days of first or second WW. Churches weren't so empty ever in the whole human history.*

The inherent weakness of mankind in face of a violent nature was never so evident. God or his son—or even the two collectively couldn't do anything to help the situation.

Summer holiday season, so very characteristic of the western civilisation, wasn't simply shortened—but the countries that had shown eagerness to benefit from the same were punished harshly by the revengeful virus through deadly second and third waves of enhanced infection and a significant spike in number of victims. And the dreaded virus was seen throwing its dark shadow on the 2020-2021 Christmas and New Year holiday season too.

> *A new sort of dark winter was imposed by the great virus on major parts of the world. A large number of people who faced movement and work-related restrictions felt discomforted; some simply descended into depression and related mental conditions.*

The dreaded Corona had stripped a large part of the mankind of normal pleasure and happiness.

* * *

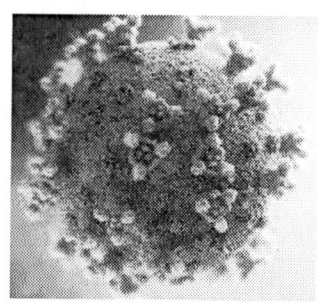

EPISODE 13

CORONA PUSHED SOME GOVERNMENTS TO ABDICATE GOVERNANCE

Coronavirus exhibited great capacity to confuse and/or imbalance some governments into abdicating responsibility for judicious governance. In Covid-19 times every government's specific responsibility was (a) to guide its people how not to fall prey to the pandemic, (b) treat and rehabilitate those infected, and (c) treat with dignity those who unfortunately fell prey to the disease. Most of the governments in the world did their best towards protecting their citizens against the dreaded pathogen by employing (a) the test, trace and isolate strategy advocated by the WHO, and (b) treat the ones needing medical attention. The efficient ones attempted to upgrade medical facilities in order to face the challenge, in addition to helping financially those rendered jobless and had lost income.

> *Several governments, however, failed to effectively discharge their constitutional duties to varying degree on account of either some inbuilt defects in their systems of governance, or due to political conflicts faced by them. In some cases, just pure incompetence, or stark insensitivity towards the basic needs of their people seemed being the main cause of non-performance, or ineffectiveness and delayed actions on their part. Disregard to scientific advice mattered a lot in most such cases.*

Major cases of such failures related to India, Brazil, and the United States of America—and in all the three cases the major cause of failure rested right at top of the governance pyramid. The Hindutva-stained government in India miserable failed even to ensure respectful last rights to Corona victims.

> *Dead bodies were disrespectfully thrown into rivers or buried in shallow sand pits in riverbeds where dogs and wild animals were seen heaping the ultimate disrespect upon them. The ugliest face of Hindutva was so exposed by the insensitive administration that was seen not even admitting its misdeeds.*

When Corona raised its ugly head in the 1st quarter of 2020, the Narendra Modi government was seen being actively engaged with (a) engineering communal riots in Delhi, (b) toppling democratically elected state governments headed by opposition parties, and (c) welcoming President Trump on a state visit. Covid-19, despite its 30th January appearance in Kerala state, was nowhere on its sensitivity screen and hence the need to prepare to safeguard its people when the pandemic struck more visibly in March 2020, wasn't visible in its list of priorities. It wanted to strengthen its case as a major world power just by claiming that soon it was going to turn into a *'Vishva Guru'* with a US dollar 5 trillion economy. Arrogance of having a brute majority in the Parliament and its ability to have subdued all the key constitutionally established institutions of the country, including the Supreme Court of India, had filled it with significant anti-people arrogance and its unpleasant expressions.

> *Indian economy was already in a bad state when Corona knocked at its door—and the government didn't know how to deal with the situation, except raising fuel costs, on one hand and reducing the common-man's income, on the other by repeatedly reducing interest rates on small deposits and other saving instruments.*

Without any planning and consultations, it imposed three weeks' long lockout with 4 hours' notice. A great majority of the population was locked up in their tiny dwellings without income and daily need provisions. The hypes-loving PM of India stated that great epic battle of Kurukshetra was won in 18 days and that Covid-19 too will be defeated through the so clamped lockdown in 21 days (the durations of its 1st phase of lockdown). There was, indeed, no need not to give time to people for securing daily need provisions as the total number of Covid-19 cases at that time was only 500 in the vast populace of 1300 million. A notice of a day or two wouldn't have damaged the situation anymore adversely.

People co-operated but they were in for the century's greatest misery as the injudiciously imposed lockout was extended three times up to middle of May. By this time over 400 million industrial labourers, daily wagers and small businessmen who had lost jobs and incomes, were under pressure from landlords to vacate their small, rented accommodations. And since they couldn't any more live with empty stomach under uncertain and stressful conditions, most of them were on road to go to their villages. Absence of transport, as buses and trains were non-functional, added to their miseries. State governments as well as the Central one ignored the large masses moving on roads on foot and on bikes—some falling prey to hunger and thirst—and numerous were crushed to death by speed loving trucks.

> *Sacred of loss of reputation, the majority blinded Central Government directed police to stop the so moving masses and the police went berserk with their sticks. People suffered a raw deal but kept moving despite being hungry, thirsty and tired.*

The insensitive administration now seemed pressurized by the disastrous situation and restarted train and bus transport in a clumsy and unplanned manner which further intensified people's misery. Left without food and water people were seen dying in trains' bathrooms and on plate-forms in an unexpectedly inhuman manner.

The government failed to assess what was coming after the three times extended lockout was lifted in mid-May, as it had turned excessively centralised and autocratic. Adequate preparations weren't made to upgrade hospitals, add new beds and ICUs in adequate number and procure testing kits, PPEs, and other necessities. Its main emphasis centred upon blaming opposition ruled state governments and cornering them on one or the other pretext. Disaster Management Act was invoked and that put all emergency powers in hands of the already imbalanced and inefficient Central Government.

When Covid-19 assumed a threatening form and number of infected people and deaths on account of the same accelerated on daily basis, people couldn't get themselves tested even against payment. The cost of getting tested in private labs was high and rules in regard to getting tested were altered at confusing pace. *Infected patients ran from one hospital to another and many died at gates of hospitals or in ambulances.* Private hospitals not only charged prohibitively high fee ranging from $ 500-1000 per day but insisted for huge advance deposits from the so stressed patients. As if it wasn't enough, dead were treated worse than animals in government hospitals. Dead bodies were stored alongside patients in hospital wards. And conflict in regard to blame apportioning grew between state governments and the Centre; the latter was seen trying to push the formers into submission by employing coercing powers bestowed on it under various provisions of the Disaster Management Act.

Death and infection numbers grew constantly in May and June 2020 and India reached the 4th spot in the world in regard to intensity of infection and deaths.

> *The publicity-loving Central Government had massive control over print and TV media—and hence, it attempted to whitewash its multilateral failures repeatedly.*

Its attempts to prop-up the nose-diving economy wasn't much of a success and the country continued to struggle on Covid-19 induced fronts for a long time. In July and August Corona went rural and there were more death than what were recorded. India's situation continued being precarious when all through September and most of October it led the world with daily reported cases of infection and deaths.

> *Mismanagement of the second wave of the pandemic in April and May 2021 exposed the inefficiency and utter insensitivity of the Indian government in most horrid ways (see episode 50 for details).*

Brazil was another case of serious mismanagement of the Covid-19 induced situations. Its autocratic President, Jair Bolsonaro, constantly conflicted with state governors as how to deal with the deadly pandemic. He opposed lockdown and called the Covid-19 virus just as a *'little flu'* and, in his daily public appearances, he showed utter contempt against the disease as well as the people who differed with his approach.

Crushing poverty and illiteracy in the country, on one hand and poor medical infrastructure, on the other brought Brazil to its knees in face of the deadly pandemic. By middle of June 2020, infections and death figures in the country left every other country behind except the USA. Dead bodies were being disposed-off in mass graves and relatives had no time even to have last glimpses of the departing souls. Observation of normal funeral rites was conspicuous by their absence.

> *The situation in the Brazilian society was truly chaotic and responsibility for the same squarely rested with the illogical operations of the county's President.*

Another case of mismanagement of the Covid-19 dictated situations was USA, the presumed Superpower of the world and its technology leader. Here, by mid-June 2020, over 1,10,000 people were dead, and the infected ones had crossed the figure of two million. It all resulted from President Trump's incompetent dealings with his technical advisors, on one hand and governors of several opposition ruled states, on the other. His political compulsions in regard to the upcoming re-election in November 2020 were other major causes of numerous failures on the Covid-19 front.

As the situation emerged by middle of the year, it seemed certain that USA was to maintain its lead in terms of losses of human lives at hands of the great pandemic during rest of the year too. The Superpower's economy too had taken a massive nose-dive.

All the three large Covid-19 victim countries continued to suffer greater thrashings at hands of the dreaded virus as the year 2020 progressed towards closure. By the 3rd week of November, US count of infections had crossed the massive mark of 12 million and over 2,50,000 American lives were lost to the dreaded pandemic. Further, the virus was surging unabatedly all over the country with daily new infections touching 2,00,000 and deaths had crossed the 2,000 a day. At the year ended these figures were seen on way to doubling. The state of California was in a strangulating grip of Corona; its hospitals were seen almost failing to take care of all the infected and sick. Medical professionals were now being forced to decide who had better chances of survival and thus apportion the facilities accordingly. The resultant damage to the American society was indeed immense.

India too had touched the total reported infections count of 9.0 million while factual numbers were much higher, Total reported deaths in India by now were touching 1,50,000, not counting those who died in villages unattended and uncared for. Brazil maintained its third position in terms of total infections count.

> *The situation in all the three countries wasn't posed for any betterment as the year came to close. Incompetent handling of the Covid-19 challenge in all the three major sufferers of the pandemic was starkly visible.*

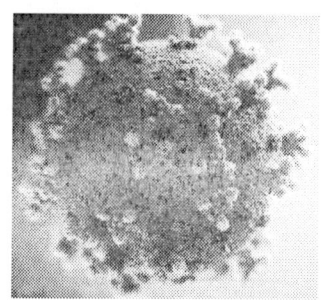

EPISODE 14

COVID TOOK A LONG RIDE ON ITS VICTIMS

Covid, as mentioned elsewhere, was a bio-agent and, possibly, it carried an overload of intelligence and selection capability. And it sure wasn't a *'tiny flu'* as was claimed by the Brazilian president Jair Bolsonaro. By middle of the Covid year 2020, it became evident that in terms of its effect on bodies of its victims, it wasn't neither tiny nor a hit and run type of pathogen.

> *Depending upon victims' age and immunity, it tended to take long residence in their bodies and caused numerous lingering adverse impacts.*

It was reported by several medical experts that Covid victims who turned negative and went home to recuperate continued to feel fatigued and weak for as long as 6-8 weeks, or even longer in some cases. About 40-45 percent of such persons complained to their doctors about the same and a large number of them returned to hospitals to seek relief. Some hospitals even opened special OPDs to deal with such patients. These sufferers of the post-Covid syndrome spoke of several complaints, in addition to persisting fatigue and general weakness—which, amongst others, included the following:

> *Respiratory distress i.e. the inability to take deep breath was most common complaint. Their lungs weren't recovering to pre-Covid capacities.*

Difficulty in walking and hence trouble of not getting back to pre-Covid normalcy of daily routine and/or job responsibilities was general refrain of most of them.

Some complained of loss of smell and taste lingering on beyond expectations. Disturbed digestion was an associated situation in some cases. Dry cough and throat irritation, in some cases, persisted as long as for six months after testing negative.

Several of them complained of a feeling of feverishness while body temperature measurement didn't confirm the condition.

Investigations on several of them confirmed existence of **'multi-organ inflammation'** which had several serious implications. Heart muscles turning weak was one of the consequences and it was reported that some young patients who attempted to get back to their previous exercise routine fell and died of heart failure.

Liver related complaints too were reported in some cases.

Mental fogginess, enhancement of forgetfulness, confusion and depression weren't uncommon in the recovering population.

Reduced hearing capacity was reported in some cases and it affected orientation in case of such victims. Facial expressions alterations were seen occurring in some cases. Cases of compromised renal function too weren't uncommon.

> *Reports of these and many other post-Covid lingering complications continued unabated all through 2020 and beyond—and it was feared that no part of the human body or related function was beyond the dreaded pathogen's capability to create trouble.*

It was proved beyond doubts that the Covid-19 wasn't a simple respiratory virus; it was much more vicious. And the medical community had a difficult job at hand to deal with it.

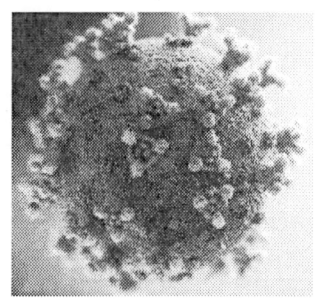

EPISODE 15

COVID-19 SPAWNED A DANGEROUS DIGITAL DIVIDE

With the spread of Covid-19 in the first quarter of 2020, covering almost the whole world, most of educational institutions closed down and students of all classes, junior as well as senior, were confined to their homes. After few months when it became clear that the virus wasn't in a hurry to disappear, management of most of such institutions resorted to conducting on-line classes for the benefit of the home quarantined students.

But all students weren't equipped to take advantage of the same; a good majority of them, particularly in the developing world, had no internet facility and couldn't also afford to buy smart phones, or avail the benefit of a laptop.

> *These have-nots not only suffered an uneven playing field but also faced the trauma of being left out because of poverty of their parents. Some of them, especially the brilliant ones, who had a great desire to do well in their studies even fell prey to depression.*

And along with them, their parents too suffered the pain of failure to adequately meet the needs of their wards.

This ***dangerous digital divide*** was witnessed by the author in India where numerous brilliant students came from economically weak families and exhibited high ambitions to do well in life. They dreamt of becoming doctors, engineers, scientists, and well-paid and powerful administrators. Their dreams were shattered by the deadly Covid-19 as it conspired with poverty to deny these ambitious youth opportunities to pursue their dreams. Under these conditions of denial and stress some of these highly ambitious youngsters turned non-communicative and suffered dejection which produced illogical thoughts and a persisting sense of being worthless, or unwanted. As a result of this greatly stressful digital divide many of these brilliant souls resorted to self-destruction and committed suicides.

> *In the first week of November 2020, a brilliant student of the prestigious Lady Shriram College, New Delhi, who came from a poor family from Telangana state, hanged herself in her home as she couldn't pursue her studies on-line in want of a smart phone and internet facilities.*

Her father, a motorcycle mechanic, couldn't provide the same despite best efforts. And college and state bureaucracies denied her benefit of a scholarship that got twined into dreadful and unsympathetic formalities. She had desired to become a high-powered administrator in the national bureaucracy.

This wasn't an isolated case where a brilliant young life was lost. There were hundreds of other such cases reported from all over the country and the insensitive Indian state, as well as the highly stratified society remained silent while the Covid-19 mocked at the situation that it had conspired to precipitate.

> *And as the dreadful pandemic continued unabatedly to collaborate with inequality, many more brilliant young lives faced a disastrous situation arising out of the dangerous digital divide.*

Many parents who couldn't pay fees and associated charges of schools and colleges withdrew their children from the education stream in a painful manner. There was a wave of school dropouts endangering future of youngsters from weaker sections of the society. Beyond India, this dangerous digital divide's dreadful impact was visible in several countries of Asia, Africa, and Latin America. Thus, Covid-19 was dreadfully discriminative.

* * *

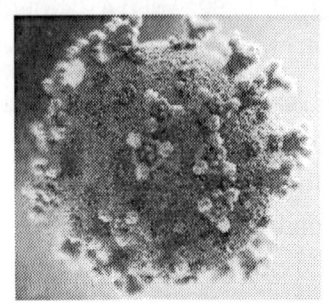

EPISODE 16

CORONAVIRUS DIVED INTO AN INTERNATIONAL CONSPIRACY

Coronavirus originated from Wuhan town in China. For weeks, the event was kept under wrap for the fear that disclosure may adversely affect trade and development.

> *It is said that China conspired with WHO not to let the deadly development to excessively worry the world, on one hand and the latter decided to mislead the world, on the other. WHO chief was either convinced or pressurised by Chinese authorities to say, early in January 2020, that the Covid-19 wasn't spreading from person to person while facts were otherwise.*

It was a misstatement of great import which worked temporarily to dull governments in several countries into insensitivity and delayed preparations to counter the danger that was moving to cause immense damage. He also pleaded with countries which thought of curtailing air travel to and fro China, not to do so because it would damage the world trade, on one hand and China's reputation, on the other.

When situation turned serious in Wuhan due to community

streaming of the infection China decided to go in for a strict lockdown, keeping millions of people within four walls of their residences for several weeks. All local transports and community activities were stopped for several weeks. It made the cat to jump out of the bag and the WHO had to cut a sorry figure. President Trump grabbed the situation and called the disease as *"Chinese Virus"*. China didn't like the designation and the controversy not only continued to grow all through the year 2020, it also splashed into 2021. The dangerous virus travelled fast around the world through unrestricted air travel and movement of tourism and trade. And by early April, almost all the over 200 countries of the world were in its grip—only severity of the disease varied in relation to inward air travel and mixing up of tourists and the trading communities.

> *It was estimated by experts that if the Chinese authorities and WHO wanted, the dreaded virus could have been contained and controlled right in Wuhan itself—and, consequently, the large loss of human life world over and the deep cut that it made on the world economy could have been avoided for the good of everyone.*

With the flaring up of the intensity of the pandemic, there arose a low intensity undercurrent in the world's diplomatic community that some countries might go to the International Court of Justice (ICJ) and claim damages from China. USA still insisted on calling the dreaded disease as **"Chinese Virus"** and China seemed somewhat unnerved by the situation which was evident from the fact that the emerging superpower reportedly had approached India and some other countries through diplomatic channels stressing that they shouldn't side with the USA in this matter.

> *As death toll mounted in various states of USA, President Trump's criticism of China grew intense and unrelenting. He alleged that the subject virus had escaped from a Wuhan virology lab and that there should be an independent international inquiry in the matter.*

Australia too directly blamed China for the great human tragedy caused by the virus world over. Prime Minister Scott Robinson aggressively asserted that China should pay compensation for the damage done to the human society. French President Macron too raised the issue. Mike Pompeo, the US Secretary of State, was direct in his attack on China and his obvious conviction in this regard seemed highly convincing.

The issue of China's complicity or culpability in regard to the spread of the Covid-19 world over continued to grow as US presidential campaign reached finality in November 2020. How the new US President weighs the issue shall determine the direction it takes in the year 2021 and whether it causes greater headache to China. And the Chinese authorities, it seemed, had assessed the damage causing potential of the lingering controversy—and in order to minimise its impact on Chinese business and polity, its diplomatic core had become activated to countering the same.

* * *

EPISODE 17

DARKEST WINTER IN HUMAN HISTORY

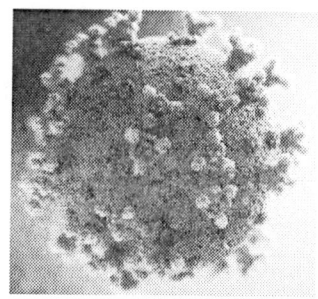

Dr Rick Bright, the senior US scientist dealing with Vaccine development program, had warned the US administration right in January 2020, about the great danger that the Coronavirus posed to its citizens and economy.

> He stressed that the country lacked tools namely—testing kits, PPEs, ventilators, hospital beds, ICUs and therapeutics needed for successfully facing the challenge thrown up by the pandemic.

Funds were also needed to initiate development of vaccines for the purpose. His pleas for speedy action in this direction were not only ignored, but he was also fired by President Trump from the job for exposing the country's unpreparedness, on one hand and the administration's insensitivity in the matter, on the other. He decided to turn into a **'whistle-blower'** and deposed before a Congressional Committee in middle of May 2020—and disclosed the truth how the Trump administration had messed-up or ignored preparations in early months of the year which were crucial for an effective fight against the virus that had turned into a pandemic. It gave a severe jolt to USA in terms of loss of human lives, the highest in the world, and deep damage to its economy.

During the deposition Dr Bright stressed that USA was not conducting enough tests to detect the disease and do the necessary follow-up actions in terms of contact tracing, identification, and isolation of the infected. The fact that there were not any tested and effective therapeutics or drugs available against the pandemic too was clarified by Dr Bright. He re-stressed that the country wasn't self-sufficient in production of the basic tools needed for effectively fighting the dreaded pandemic and that the opening up of businesses and industry in a hurry, without adequate preparations and caution, ran the danger of eruption of unmanageable surges of the deadly disease. These combined with the normal upturns of usual flu infections in the next fall season could, as per Dr Bright's assertion, turn into the **'Darkest Winter'** in modern US history. And the disaster, in fact, happened.

He added that *'time was running out for America'* since it wasn't yet ready for facing the virulent nature's challenge. The superpower's preparations, in Dr Bright's opinion, looked like headless chickens running around aimlessly. It didn't have even enough numbers of swabs, the simplest need for testing the infected or suspected cases of infection. USA depended upon imports for every item/tool needed for a sustained fight against Coronavirus pandemic.

He also elaborated that arrival of vaccine against the Covid-19 pandemic was still 12 to 18 months away. And production of adequate dosages of vaccine and distribution of the same to all who needed the same in the whole world needed great efforts and organisation.

The Covid-19 is a new virus. Human body didn't know it. The whole challenge was new, and the dreaded virus was here to stay. And the world might take up to three years to get rid of it. The virus might even turn endemic. People will need to learn to live with it through proper sanitation, social distancing, and necessary behavioural alterations. An effective vaccine will be, as of today, the only effective option.

> *President Trump, after Dr Bright's deposition tried to belittle the well-established expert. He called Dr Bright a disgruntled employee. Dr Bright had also opposed the President's attempts to promote the untested hydroxy chloroquine as a cure for the pandemic. It was added that no untested and/ or anecdotal input needed to be pushed as a cure.*

Dr Bright's courage received widespread appreciation from scientific community as well as the general public while it added to President Trump's difficulties in dealing with the situation arising out of mishandled pandemic.

> *Dr Bright's observations, though made specifically in context of American situation, had larger implication for the world community threatened by the pandemic.*

His predictions and fears, in fact, turned true right towards end of the pandemic year 2020 when whole the US was crushed by an intense wave of the vicious virus. Daily reported infections' count had crossed 2,00,000 peak and over 2,000 Americans lost their lives every day. Soon after, these figures of damage to the American society had doubled. And with enhanced hospital admissions and chaotic situation in the state of California, the superpower's medical infrastructure had felt greatly overwhelmed. As the Covid year 2020 gave way to 2021 the **'Dark Winter'** was right there, and its shadow had turned the Christmas/ New Year holiday season into a hugely disappointing occasion for Americans.

In addition, the whole Europe too had experienced a truly **'Dark Winter'** as a vicious second (or a third one at places) wave of the deadly pandemic had crushed businesses and industry, especially the travel, tourism, and associated hospitality sector, into a complex mess. Western world's superior technological status hadn't helped in any manner *in encountering the disastrous situation.*

* * *

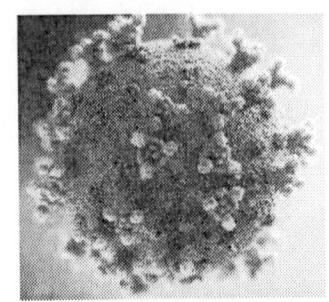

EPISODE 18

DIFFERENT APPROACHES EMPLOYED AGAINST CORONAVIRUS

All the over 200 countries that suffered significant damages at hands of the Coronavirus didn't employ same strategy to fight this invisible enemy. As a result, some suffered more than others. While some succeeded brilliantly, others went through lingering pains and huge loss of human lives. There were basically three types of approaches depending upon how countries listened to and/or responded to scientific advice, home-grown or that from the WHO—and results in terms of deaths and the duration of misery dictated by Covid-19, varied significantly.

> *Good blending of politics and science was seen being an important factor.*

Coronavirus was either a product of nature's erratic behaviour or some human-beings' deliberate mischief. Whatsoever the fact, it turned into an unexpectedly great challenge to the humanity. In most cases countries were caught hugely unprepared for the massive challenge posed by the invisible enemy.

> *Out of the multitude of countries Taiwan, Hong-Kong, South Korea, Vietnam, New Zealand, Sri Lanka and to an extent Singapore seemed to have done a relatively better job of dealing with the pandemic. In addition to listening to their respective scientific and medical experts, some cultural factors too seemed to have contributed to the outcome.*

They performed better than others in the fight against the dreaded pandemic in terms of loss of human life, on one hand, and damage to economy, on the other.

Taiwan had quickly grasped the challenge and the direction from where the wave of the great evil was coming. Right in January 2020 when the Covid-19 raised its ugly head in Wuhan (just across the narrow sea that separated it from the mainland China) it curtailed and then fully blocked the inflow of air passengers from mainland China. Thus, firstly an unmanageable load of the pathogen couldn't enter the island country—and then the government (**headed by economists and technologists**) effectively implemented the testing, tracking and isolation exercise on a massive scale. The result was that not more than half a dozen deaths could occur in the well-integrated and literate population.

> *Additionally, it was Taiwan that informed WHO that the disease was spreading from human to human while the latter, sometime earlier, had asserted otherwise.*

South Korea, located just north of the mainland China, was slightly less swift in blocking the inflow of critical load of virus because its economic interactions with the Covid-19 originating country were much closer and more intense than those of Taiwan. But the government here went for a massive testing of those returning from China and followed up with equally intensive contacts tracing and isolation. Like Taiwan, it didn't opt for oppressive lockdown and managed to keep the damage low to its economy as well human lives were saved in a brilliant manner. It wasn't short of PPEs for its public as well as the frontline workers in its hospitals and/or isolation facilities. By end of April 2020, South Korea had declared that there were no more domestically erupting cases of the pandemic in the country—and the ones arriving in through air travellers were being dealt with suitably. It was indeed a brilliant performance considering the small nation's close vicinity with the country where from the deadly pandemic had originated.

> *In addition, the persistent pathogen made several attempts to surge and resurge and all of these were brilliantly resisted by the technologically and administratively superior establishment.*

Singapore's situation was a lot more different. Being an air travel hub and receiving a large incoming Chinese traffic, it received a heavy load of infection right in January and February 2020, but it managed the situation quite well through strict checking at the airport and other entry points, intensive testing and isolation of those found infected—and also through effective contact tracings. It managed the situation without lockout and wasn't short of hospital facilities and there was no hue and cry for PPEs and other essentials needed for fighting through the situation. Soon after the situation came under control, many its own citizens, primarily students and businessmen, returned from UK and USA when situation deteriorated in the West. This too was managed without imposing a crippling lockdown. But by middle of April 2020, its migrant workers (primarily those from India and Bangladesh) living in crowded dorms came under growing infection—and consequently a limited but strict lockdown was then imposed to control the tricky situation. Finally, the efficiently run country escaped crippling damages at hands of the dreaded pandemic. Besides, it successfully conducted a general election right in middle of the challenging situation.

Three other Asian countries namely Vietnam, New Zealand and Australia made a smart operation in their fight against Covid-19 pandemic despite proximity to China. They managed well the resurgences that occurred in July and August and even later.

In Europe, Germany, a country of 83 million people had initially employed a good politics and science-based strategy to face and fight the dangerous disease which, by now, had crippled Italy, Spain and France a great deal. It conducted a large number of tests and followed each infected person through isolation and contacts tracing. And its medical infrastructure was efficient and fast responding. There wasn't any shortage of PPEs or other facilities for its front-line staff who took care of the suspected and infected people. Just with a relatively much lower damage to human life compared to what was suffered by three South European nations, it tackled the situation efficiently. But against the second wave that over-ran the whole Europe in November and December it was seen being much less effective.

On the other hand, several countries including the developed ones, failed to timely employ an effective mix of politics and science-based strategy, primarily delaying measures to curtail/stop inflow of infection from China (and also from other destinations) through air travel—and then found that they weren't suitably ready to face the challenge of the dreaded pathogen's assault. Their medical infrastructure was not ready with enough hospital beds, ICUs and needed PPEs and ventilators. They also hesitated or dithered in clamping down the essential lockdowns for ensuring physical or social distancing. These countries primarily included Italy, Spain, France, UK, and USA. In case of the latter politics seemed actively conflicting with science and the result was disastrous.

> *Former President Barak Obama while commenting upon the situation in early May, 2020, said that US handling of the Covid-19 pandemic was a chaotic disaster.*

And then there were the so-called developing countries like India, Pakistan, Iran, Brazil, South Africa, and numerous others **where politics and police power combined to first avoid taking right decisions and substantially acted against public interest, especially that of the poor and unemployed.**

> For most of these countries law and order was more important than protecting the masses.

Turkey despite its autocratic government managed in a much more matured manner. Others were seen busy blame apportioning to either opposition parties, or on to some religious groups. India's approach of a strict lockdown without much thought and preparations was particularly damaging to interests of migrant workers and poor masses. They suffered a great deal.

> And the second wave of the virus in April/May 2021 knocked the bottom off India's assertion that it had done better than several developed countries in the world in its efforts to counter the pandemic.

South American countries like Brazil, Peru and several others performed worst in the world in safeguarding the masses against the deadly pandemic.

* * *

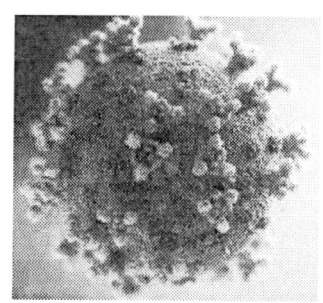

EPISODE 19

EUROPE STRUGGLED TO PROPEL ITS STALLED ECONOMY

At end of the 3rd week of May 2020, Germany, and France, the two largest economies of Europe, decided to create an over half-a-trillion Euro stimulus fund and after 3-4 meetings, virtual and otherwise, a 750 billion package—part grant and rest loan was approved in July 2020 for kick-starting the Covid-19 stalled economies. In the 27 members grouping, initially there was no consensus in this regard. Austria, Denmark, Sweden, Finland, and several other members of the Union did not seem to agree with the approach. The differences related to whether the assistance extended to the Corona-dented countries of the South was to be a loan or an outright grant.

> *The package supporting countries wanted EU to work collectively, reduce its dependence on imports of critical items and technologies, especially from China. They argued that EU should develop its own 5G technology and be self-sufficient regarding its needs for artificial intelligence (AI) etc. The need to do so in regard to critical medical requirements had been stressed. It was also stressed that EU should come up as a 3rd superpower in addition to USA and China, rather than side in one or the other way.*

By this time, Germany had opened up a large part of its economy. The iconic Bundesliga had gone ahead to practice and play football in empty stadia. Baltic nations were ahead than the central and southern Europe in the massive struggle to free their economies from Corona pandemic's strangulating grip.

Spain too had opened up its industry and businesses except in major cities, namely Madrid and Barcelona. Italy, that had suffered maximum damage at hands of the deadly pandemic, too had taken initial steps to free itself from the harsh restrictions that it had endured for the past over two months. Keeping in view the needs of its travel and tourism industry, Italy announced to resume air travel from early June. It didn't want to lose summer months when Italian beaches come alive with hordes of tourists from all over Europe. Spain, France, and other coastal countries that had waited for the great opportunity to wash off the strains imposed by the great pandemic that had crippled the southern Europe's economy, too were keen to open for the summer.

> *By middle of June 2020, travel restrictions in most of the European countries were lifted but the tourists didn't rush in. They were careful on one end and fearful of the resurge of the pandemic, on the other. Spain and UK still struggled with the need for visitors to quarantine or not to quarantine which limited benefits of opening-up of the economy. With restrictions of social distancing still in place in several countries, businesses like restaurants and bars operated only with limited attendance. Some cinema companies experimented with drive-in operations.*

Overall, it seemed that the opening-up of the economy was going to be a long-drawn effort which extended well beyond middle of the business unlucky year 2020.

By 4th week of June 2020, the tourism dependent nations of Europe—Italy, Spain, France, and Greece in particular, were in a hurry to salvage what was left of the summer season—and by end of the month, movement of tourism related visitors was fully restored though people seemed reluctant to hurry up. One major worry was USA where resurgence of the Covid-19 was in full bloom and without tourists from across the Atlantic the summer of Europe remained only half activated.

> *Despite doing its best, Europe couldn't savage much of the tourism business and on account of (a) obvious hurry in opening-up of tourism related travel and entertainment, and (b) governments' inability to restrain people from over mixing at beaches and in restaurants and bars, led to re-activation of virus in countries such as Spain, Portugal, France, France, Belgium, Germany etc. amongst others, to an extent that by end of July 2020, the continent was on verge of a second wave. It was relocking up in bits and pieces.*

It seemed that the non-forgiving virus was punishing Europe for the openness and entertainment loving nature of its society. Economy of various European countries (measured as GDP) was reported to have suffered in the range of 10-20 percent due to the great pandemic.

In September and October, resurgence of virus gathered further speed, primarily due to youngsters gathering in restaurants and bars and on beaches and also due to the unrestricted flow of alcohol, thus ruining all hopes of economic recovery in the current year.

In second and third weeks of October Europe, in fact, had turned into an epicentre of Corona infections. Belgium openly admitted that it was not capable of facing the tsunami of Covid-19 infections. Spain declared health emergency and several of its business and tourism centres were put under lockdowns. France imposed night curfew in several of its large cities, including capital Paris and restricted timings of opening and closing of bars and restaurants in an effort to contain the second wave of the dreaded virus. Italy too imposed restriction on movement of people and usage of face masks was made compulsory. UK, Germany, Netherland, amongst others, too suffered a great deal during the surging waves of the dreaded virus.

> *At several places in Europe people protested against the restrictions imposed by different governments. In fact, Europe's reputation as a developed and resourceful region was dented on account of its failure to prevent the great resurgence of the dreaded virus.*

Europe's struggle against the second wave of Corona turned grim every day as October drew towards end and November brought no respite. France faced a national crisis as more than 50 percent of hospital beds were filled by Covid patients and several medical professionals pondered over leaving their jobs for fear of being struck by the dreaded virus. French government was in a quandary as what new restrictions to impose in order to deal with the grave situation and also allow the already crippled economy to avoid further damages. Also, citizens in several countries were seen protesting more vigorously against life and work crippling restrictions. Intra-Europe travel became significantly restrictive in light of most countries demanding a negative test report from travellers or warned them of quarantine at destinations. It was now widely assumed that only arrival of some effective vaccine and its easy availability was the only way to solve the problem of people's collective interactions which for business and industry were an absolutely necessity. Europe's struggle against the deadly pandemic extended well beyond the Covid-19 year 2020 and first half of the year 2021 too saw little relief despite arrival of several vaccines as UK, South African and Brazilian variants continued to create deep chaos.

* * *

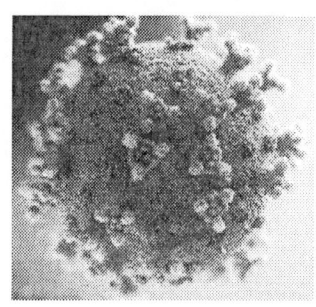

EPISODE 20

SOME GREAT HEIGHTS OF CORONA CARNAGE

In the first six months of the Corona year 2020, the Covid-19 pandemic achieved two great heights during its cyclonic spread.

One: *It covered the whole world i.e., all the six continents at a break-neck speed. Starting from Wuhan in China, first it moved to some East Asian and South European countries right in February and March. Soon, it jumped to North America—and then leisurely covered all countries in Asia, Africa, rest of Europe and South America. First, it travelled with air passengers and during its second leg moved by all means of transport employed by tourism and business travellers. It showed preference for public transport and congested spaces of hotels, bars, gyms, restaurants, and malls etc.*

Two: *Though it killed furiously all through its world-wide rampage, the second great milestone was achieved by end of June 2020, i.e., on completion of the first six months of its cyclonic march when it reached the 10 million infections mark and half a million deaths collectively world over. Of these, USA alone accounted for over 1,25,000 deaths and over 2.5 million infections. Brazil in South America, where its President Jair Bolsonaro had called the great pandemic a* ***'little flu'*** *received the world's second harshest drubbing with over 60,000 deaths and over a million infections. In both the cases, i.e., USA as well as Brazil, autocratic governance was largely responsible for the great suffering that fell upon people.*

USA was suffering a great resurge of the virus in June 2020 after the Trump administration's hurried and unwise opening-up of the economy in May and June. Now over 30 of its states were in a grip of resurging virus, daily count of new infections reaching over 60,000 by the first week of July. Consequently, the medical facilities in the country were hugely stressed. *And the country's most respected expert Dr Anthony Fauci warned that if serious measures weren't taken, the country could lose another 1,00,000 lives in next few months. For the folly of administration, the great Superpower was on the mat for a second time.*

USA, the world's dominant Superpower had taken the great virus' February 2020 arrival a little lightly. The Trump administration was busy cutting deals and enjoying foreign visits rather than preparing to face the emerging pandemic. Its public health facilities were in a mess and there was a wide-spread shortage of essentials like PPE kits, masks, and ventilators. By mid-July 2020, further new heights were scaled by the great virus as the worldwide count of infections had reached 13.1 million. USA led the world with over 3.3 million infections and 1,35,000 deaths. Brazil followed with over 2 million infections and an unexpectedly large numbers of mortalities. And India touched a million mark in terms of confirmed infections while the factual figure was expected to be much higher. Its official mortalities figure lingered on just around 30,000.

> *Surge and/or resurge by the virus was establishing new record at mid-July as it had over 35 US states under its grip, forcing closure of hurriedly opened-up businesses. Florida, Texas, and California were punished for the un-disciplined behaviour of state administrations and the people who had crowded beaches, bars, restaurants, and other closed-door and congested spaces were thrashed severely.*

By end of July 2020, confirmed world-wide infections of the deadly virus had climbed to over 17.1 million. Reported deaths rose to over 7,00,000 of which the share of USA alone was over 1,50,000. And Brazil seemed running at heals of the great Superpower with over 2.6 million reported infections and over 90,000 deaths, while actual figures were claimed being much higher by informed sources. In terms of reported deaths, Mexico with a figure of over 46,000 deaths had occupied the third place leaving UK behind. India lingered on at the fifth place in terms of deaths, with a figure of just 37,000 while its confirmed cases of infections had crossed 1.7 million.

The powerful virus had forced Europe to stop in its tracks as it attempted to, at least partially, salvage the summer tourist season—and was pushed into now haltingly facing the second wave of infections. Europe and the new world were not alone in this precarious situation as it was reported by the WHO that at end of July 2020 over three billion people, collectively in over 70 countries of the world were under varied degrees of lockdown. Australia had declared a state of disaster in Victoria on account of almost out of control surge of the deadly virus.

By 10th August 2020, the total reported infections in the world totalled over 20 million—USA led with over five million while Brazil and India crossed three and two million cases respectively. In terms of deaths, Brazil now crossed the 1,00,000 threshold and India was well over 42,000 lives lost. Some experts claimed that by end of the year USA could lose another 1,00,000 lives over and above the 1,65,000 already in graves (and the prediction had, indeed, come true). In the month of August and September, for over several weeks (3rd August through whole September), India led the world with highest reported daily infections (ranging between 50,000 to 90,000) and in terms of total reported deaths over 80,000 had left Mexico far behind—and its total infections count too had crossed the level of 5.0 million. *Experts now feared that by end of the year 2020, India might leave USA behind in terms of reported infections and, possibly, in terms of total reported deaths too (the fear didn't really come true).* Total worldwide reported death toll on account of the Covid-19 had crossed a million mark by middle of September 2020 and the global total of reported infections now stood over 30 million. By end of September

2020 the death toll in USA was well over 2,00,000 mark and the revengeful virus had struck down the boisterous *President Trump* *who had to run to a hospital while his whole re-election campaign team was mauled into limited action. Trump now faced an uncertain future. His subsequent defeat in November 2020 partly resulted out of his administration's mishandling of the great pandemic.*

On the European front, the great virus now resurged unabated. Spain, France, UK, and Russia were on the mat while rest of the continent struggled to stay upright.

India continued to lead the world in terms of daily confirmed infections and daily count of deaths; soon it was expected to leave Brazil behind in terms of lives lost on account of the deadly virus. By middle of November 2020, USA had lost over 2,50,000 lives to the dreaded virus—and as feared it now faced a *'Dark Winter'* as the year progressed towards a sad closure. The highly mobile and skilful virus, in view of the author, was destined to achieve several other great heights before it decided to leave mankind at some peace, possibly in the second half of 2021 when vaccines were expected to offer an effective counter.

Later in April/May 2021 Corona achieved the greatest height in terms of daily infections of over 4,00,000 and daily reported deaths of over 4000 for a single country during India's disastrous second wave. And actual figures were several times higher than the reported ones.

* * *

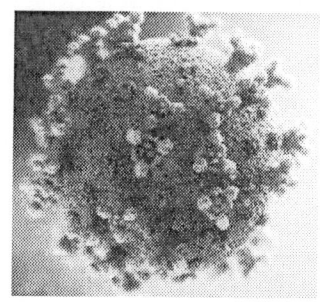

EPISODE 21

FULMINATIONS OF PRESIDENT TRUMP

All through January and February 2020, President Trump underplayed the threat of the Coronavirus. He ignored White House advisors' reports that highlighted damages likely to be inflicted upon the American people and the superpower's economy. In February, he was busy with his India visit, praising his old friend Narendra Modi, learning to say Namaste instead of handshaking to avoid infection—and staged photo opportunities at Agra with the great monument of Taj in the background.

On way home from India in the 'Air-force One' too he underplayed the danger of Coronavirus to the US society and its economy. He gave the impression, covert and/or overt, that America was strong and well-prepared to face the Corona challenge, while the facts were clearly opposite. Events that unfolded in the months of March and April 2020 proved that the US medical infrastructure was in a bad shape; there weren't enough beds and ICUs to face the situation and not even the basic requirements such as face masks and PPEs were available in adequate numbers. And ventilators needed for care of critical patients either didn't exist or were not in operative form. Even manufactures of such devices in the country were not able to stage a sudden surge of output. Finally, when situation deteriorated, scramble for import of these essentials was the only option. Since the pandemic had spread to over 200 countries in the world, supplies weren't easily available. President Trump and numerous state Governors were seen engaged in a game of blame apportioning in regard to the availability and procurement of PPEs and other essential tools needed for an effective fight against the invisible enemy. The great superpower was found with its pants down and exposed its utter vulnerability to the plundering of the pandemic.

At one stage, President Trump had praised China for handling the new disease—but soon after he blamed the emerging superpower for not being transparent with numbers of the dreaded Corona's victims in the country and in regard to origin of the pathogen. Same deviant tendency the President was displayed in praise of WTO (at one stage) and subsequently berating its chief for having favoured China, on one hand and then misguiding the world about restricting and/or stoppage of air travel to and from China, on the other.

At home, the President was seen being at loggerheads (a) with state Governors, on one hand and (b) with medical experts who wanted him to take prompt action towards arranging for basic necessities for hospitals for preventing a surge of the pandemic, on the other.

The President also differed with experts and state Governors regarding the timing and length of lockdown and the need and quantum of support/recovery package to the vulnerable sections of industry and businesses, as well as, to those rendered unemployed due to lockdown. He underplayed the need for aggressive testing of people, isolation of those found positive and their contacts tracing that were needed for containing the massive ingress of the dreaded virus. *His daily press briefings regarding the Pandemic's spread and intensity were a spectacle of contradictions and unscientific utterances.*

The President was also seen underplaying the need for testing facilities and needed availability of PPE kits etc for the purpose of effectively countering the Pandemic. And then, he wasn't comfortable with surging data of infected people and also deaths in the month of March and April 2020. The metropolis of New York suffered maximum infections and deaths—and its Governor Cuomo was seen complaining about the visible deficiencies in the fight against the dreaded Covid-19, all through the period that saw disturbing sure of infections and deaths of people.

> *About the need for general public to cover faces and put on a simple device like a mask too, President Trump often seemed confusing the people; he himself was always seen without wearing a face mask.*

Dr Anthony Fauci of the CDC, a renowned medical expert on communicable diseases, was seen running the risk of being fired by the President for his differing views as how to deal with the dreaded virus. Several other medical experts/virologists too politely and skilfully differed with the President but towards end of April 2020, US media was seen aggressively questioning the President's inconsistent and unscientific approach towards fighting the dreaded virus.

Mounting US figures of infected people (over 9,00,000) and over 53,000 deaths by the end of April 2020, highest in the world, and the spread of the pandemic to almost all the 50 states unnerved the President; his unease was visible on his face.

> *In one customary White House press briefing he suggested use/ injecting detergents into patients' bodies for controlling the devastating pandemic. This, as expected, didn't go well with the scientific community—and it led to more open and aggressive criticism of the impulsive President. An obviously unnerved President proceeded to temporarily suspend the usual daily White House press briefings.*

By middle of April 2020, the President had started talking about reopening of the lock-downed and a resultant nose-diving economy.

Unemployment rate and those who applied for assistance rose to over 22 million by this time. It sharpened the President's itch for opening up the lock-downed economy and businesses. On this issue too he differed with medical experts, as well as state Governors and economic experts.

By the 3rd week of April 2020, the President seemed to have grown impatient with the national lockdown and the damage that it had done to the economy. Now, he was seen encouraging his followers in opposition ruled states to agitate for opening of the economy. The possibility of losing the election in November was making the US President obviously nervous.

Commentators on US approach towards fighting the Corona pandemic and the resultant situation, economic and otherwise, arising out of it, became aggressively critical of the President—and some even went to say that the US handling of the situation was akin to what would have come from a resource starved third world country.

> *The most striking observation in this regard came from former President Barak Obama in early May when he said that handling of the Covid-19 pandemic in USA was a chaotic disaster.*

At one stage President Trump also attempted to lay blame for the devastating run of the Corona pandemic all over the world on to the WHO and suspended US aid to it. Experts saw this too as an impulsive action of an unnerved President. USA was now seen progressively losing world leadership that was urgently needed in this challenging situation for fighting the great pandemic.

Early in the month of May 2020, most US states had started selectively lifting the lockdown and opening up the economy. Some states were seen going faster in the process and freed even malls, beeches, parks, and games arenas while others limited initial effort to small businesses and shops. All the state authorities, however, exhibited uncertainty and apprehension about possible resurgences or second wave of the dreaded diseases on easing of restrictions. By this time US deaths had climbed to over 65,000 and infected persons count crossed a million mark.

All through the second and third week of May 2020, the number of total infections and deaths caused in US by the pandemic continued to rise. Over 1,00,000 persons had perished by end of the 3rd week of May 2020 and it wasn't difficult to assume that by end of the 3rd quarter of the year the figure might double or go even higher.

Confrontation between the ruling Republicans and opponent Democrats has been escalating progressively. Democrats' dominated Congress passed a resolution approving a 3 trillion stimulus package designed to activate working of businesses and industries that attempted to reopen in the past few weeks. It was, however, expected to be blocked by the Senate dominated by the ruling party.

> *During a virtual function of newly passing graduates, former President Barak Obama commented that no one in the Trump administration seemed to know that he or she was in-charge of anything.*

President Trump had been advocating for opening-up of schools in September arguing that children were almost immune to Covid-19. In first week of August 2020, FB and Twitter deleted President's postings on these social media as they were seen unscientific and misleading. For several months President Trump had been making misleading comments about his administration's failure to control surging spread of the pandemic.

> *His chances in the November re-election by now seemed severely dented on account of his Covid-19 related fulminations.*

These and numerous other inconsistencies on part of President Trump led to his losing the re-election battle in November 2020.

* * *

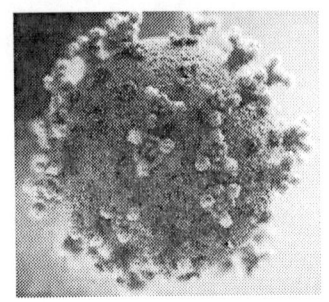

EPISODE 22

HOW SHOULD WORLD CHANGE FOR SAFER FUTURE?

Covid-19 pandemic offered several lesions to the mankind for its safer and healthier future. It has been, indeed, a cruel agent of the nature, yet in its ruthlessness were hidden numerous instructions as how damage in future from similar agents could be avoided or minimised.

> *First of all, mankind should shun, or at least minimise, needless elements of globalisation because on account of the inherent negative human nature, dependence on others beyond a certain level is harmful in the long-term for the welfare of the human race.*

One's dependence on others should be such, or of such a degree, that when needed self-reliance could be attained just in a jerk or in such a short time that lasting damage of any type is avoided. At the Covid-19 time most of the countries which suffered heavy damage in terms of infections and deaths were excessively dependent on China for a variety of supplies and services.

Travel, especially the air travel, is one of the major components of globalisation. It has disastrous influence on our living environment through toxic emissions and consequent climate alterations. In fact, any mode of transport that burned fossil fuel should be minimised for the mankind's bright future. People should be encouraged, or even rewarded for shunning cars and taking to biking and/or the on-foot travel; it will improve health as well as prosperity, on one hand and almost eliminate pathogens fast riding with us, on the other.

> *Tourism, especially as an entertainment or enjoyment input, is potentially an activity of uncertain value addition when compared to the unsustainable load that it puts on the environment. It encourages undesirable practices and greater intermingling or interactions of human beings that are bound to spread pathogens and/or unhealthy social practices.*

However, tourism when undertaken for attaining knowledge or erudition is a healthy and desirable activity.

The Corona pandemic has also instructed mankind for greater investments in health infrastructure which is any day more important than investments in travel, tourism and/or entertainment infrastructures.

> *Covid-19 also instructs mankind to depend on science and technology for governance policies and decisions than on dictatorial and/or autocratic political formations presently overtaking major parts of the world.*

Police and paramilitary forces in hands of dictators and autocrats end up being misused against the very people that they are originally designed to protect. This was seen happening in several countries in the Covid-19 times when authoritarianism spurted in governance as dealing with the pandemic had made it easier to justify tighter controls on public affairs and on people's lives.

Speed of action and/or timely measures are better alternatives to deal with disasters and calamities than simple strict and unplanned lockdowns.

> *The modern approach to urbanisation and industrialisation which puts too many people (migrants and industrial workers) in congested dwellings needs to be minimised or given up entirely. Reduced globalisation and more dependence on localisation and resultant self-reliance will help in this regard.*
>
> *The Corona pandemic also went on to suggest that some communities eagerly making a meal of wild animals were needed to be discouraged in order to avoid pathogens jumping from wild to humans.*

For its own safety mankind needs to increasingly go vegetarian in its food habits. Through actively planned efforts it should minimise interfering with the nature, especially the wild animals' world.

Corona also went ahead to suggest that high density human habitations such as slums and ghettoes were a clear invitation to disaster at hands of a variety of pathogens. There, in fact, is no justification for crowding millions of people in unmanageable urban habitations.

> *Further, there are numerous other hidden messages from the Corona stressed situations which mankind need to decode and ponder upon for ensuring its own safety in future.*

* * *

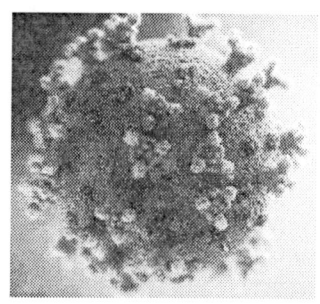

EPISODE 23

INDIAN DIASPORA AND DOMESTIC MIGRANT WORKERS

Indian government displayed a discriminative response to the plight of domestic migrant workers and the Indian diaspora during the post-lockdown 2.0 in the first week of May 2020. The domestic migrant workers who couldn't walk to their homes at distant places had remained holed up at their workplaces, hungry and neglected by governments—their home states as well as the ones for which they had worked. These workers had expected that after the lockdown 2.0 which had ended on 3rd May 2020, buses and trains would restart—but when it didn't come through by end of the first week of May, they became desperate and huge protests emerged at Chennai, Hyderabad, Mumbai, Ahmedabad, and Surat. Police, as usual, resorted to use of force resulting in uncontrolled chaos; the central government had to give-in and announced that trains (point-to-point) shall resume and take the distort worker's home. Some trains were to move from Kerala and Telangana in the first week, but arrangements were chaotic—and poor migrants who had not been paid for months, were forced to pay for the train fares by collecting money through borrowing and begging.

> *The Indian Railways that had just contributed to the PM relief fund Rs. 151 crores was insensitive to migrants' miseries. Government, central or state, wouldn't have become bankrupt by absorbing this minuscule expenditure.*

It showed governments' long prevailing insensitivity to the plight of desperate and destitute workers. Having not been allowed to get into right trains or being unable to pay for the train tickets, thousands of workers took to walking on foot to their homes thousands of miles away. Hungry, thirsty, and sick of months long deprivation, some of them fell dead on roads or were crushed by fast moving vehicles—and no one from central and/or local governments bothered to look at them.

> *Police treated them with shower of sticks as the scene on the roads picked up by some TV channels was inconvenient for the GOI that often played impressive song and dance stories for welfare of people. Distressed migrants moved to Railway tracks to avoid beatings by the police.*

Only some villagers helped the hungry and tired. It proved beyond doubt that the NDA government in Delhi that often talked proudly of India becoming a $ five trillion economy as result of its efficient handling of things, economic and otherwise, was totally blind towards the misery of the commonest of the common men and women of India. However, the plight of the migrant workers waking on roads and some falling dead wasn't missed by some TV channels, including some foreign ones. And the government in Delhi behaved as if nothing was wrong and that the Covid-19 management including the great Indian lockouts, were just going great. Government spokesmen, long habituated of indulging in self-praise, claimed that the world had praised the great Indian lockouts that kept the infection low. Facts, however, were painfully otherwise.

> *Some 16 migrant labours who were walking along the rail tracks between Jalana and Aurangabad (in Maharashtra state), tired and exhausted, they fell asleep on the tracks and were crushed by a goods train.*

Though they were denied a train to go home but their dead bodies, cut into pieces, were now carried away by a train. And in a deadly contrast, officials went to visit the accident spot by a state plane. And the plight of pregnant women giving birth on roads and rail tracks was indeed poignant. Government operations were seen in worst form in the over 75 years' long history of independent India.

> *Even during the partition necessitated migration (when state resources were not even five percent of the 2020, government that had claimed itself as the 5th largest economy of the world) such state insensitivity was never witnessed.*

On the other hand, the diaspora friendly government in India announced in the first week of May 2020 that it would organise over a hundred Air India flights to bring home several hundred thousands of Indians stranded in Europe and Middle East. Even some Indian Navy ships were ordered to collect such persons from Middle East and Maldivian ports. The discriminative approach was there for everyone to see.

* * *

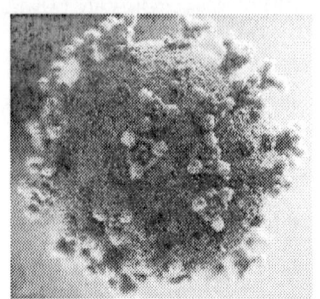

EPISODE 24

INDIAN LOCKDOWN SUCCUMBED TO PUBLIC PROTESTS

> *Lockdown in India was first imposed on 24th of March 2020. It was done without much thought and planning for welfare of poor people. Restrictions on movements of people were imposed just at 4 hours' notice and, consequently, millions of daily wagers and migrant workers were stranded away from their homes without provision of earnings, food and shelter.*

Even millions of middle-class families were left without provisions needed for daily life maintenance. Trains and road transport was discontinued in a knee-jerk impulse while the air travel that brought the Pandemic's infection to the country was allowed to continue unrestricted for several days.

The jobless and homeless workers so held up in industrial hubs of the country suffered hunger and deprivation for several weeks. Dictated by the situation created by the government's knee-jerk decision thousands of them walked long distances to their villages carrying small loads of their belongings as head loads. Ladies carried small children as additional load and suffered hunger, thirst, and tiredness in truly inhuman situations.

> *Many fell dead on the way to home with no one to weep for them. But by middle of April, patience and tolerance of those still held up at their work locations, had given way to protests and agitations—and scenes so generated, amongst others, at Chennai, Mumbai, Surat and Hyderabad rattled several state governments. Only Chennai was reported to holding over 200,000 migrant labours desperate to go home.*

Desperation of migrants was highlighted by one incidence at Indore in central India where over a dozen of them were caught travelling to UP inside a rotating cement container, in a truly life-threatening condition. There could have been no better evidence of desperation on part of the migrant workers. They were prepared to risk death for reaching home—and many of them paid for such a desperation right on risky Indian roads.

Additionally, several thousand students held up at Kota in Rajasthan when hostels closed and their safety and security turned into a risk, added another element to the precarious human situation. Several state governments were forced to send fleets of buses to bring home the so held-up students from Kota. Now, by end of April 2020, Government of India was compelled to start trains to take the lockdown stranded migrant workers to their respective home states. Point to point trains such as Hyderabad to Jharkhand and others from Kerala, Mumbai, and several other places to destinations in UP, Bihar, Bengal and Orissa were arranged. And in the meantime, precisely on May 1, 2020, the labour's day, the dreaded lockdown was further extended for two more weeks which was called lockdown 3.0.

By implication of what happened at end of April 2020 i.e., at end of the second phase of lockdown, the unplanned and anti-poor nature of the India's much touted about lockdown were unmasked for everyone to see. But the Government of India that was elected with huge majority, just two years earlier, had no words of regret for its folly, nor it showed any sympathy or effort for relief to the poor who suffered so greatly.

> *Migrant workers received no meaningful help from state governments who seemed confused whether to send them home or retain for eventual restart of commercial activities. Contractors and businesses did not pay them April salaries. Disheartened and hungry, a greater mass of the workers was seen on roads walking on foot or pushing rickety bikes in direction of their home states. Since the scene didn't suit the government, police were told to push the migrant workers away or persuade them to stay wherever they happened to be; dismayed workers now moved to Railway tracks to avoid beatings by the police.*

Confused by the situation, state governments asked for more trains to take the workers home and some progress in this direction was seen only by middle of May 2020.

Now, further extension of the lockdown called lockdown 4.0 was announced and a confusing Rs. 20 lakh crores of aid package to businesses and industry too was declared. The lockdown 4.0 and opening-up of businesses and industry was supposed to move together. The NDA government expected to stimulate the supply side of economy which, in principle, looked like a faulty move. It was seen based more on politics than needs of the collapsed economy. The mishandled Indian economy suffered a 23.9 percent fall in the second quarter of the financial year 2020-21.

* * *

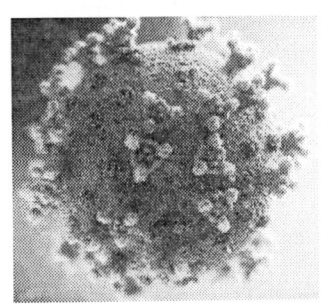

EPISODE 25

LOCKDOWNS AND INEVITABILITY OF SECOND WAVE

Lockdowns are a measure of limited or uncertain merit in relation to controlling the Corona pandemic. Its demerits or negative impacts on the economic, social, cultural, emotional, and even psychological fabric of the impacted society are immense.

> *Corona is an intelligent bio-agent. It knows when to lie low and when to surge and resurge with vengeance. It coordinates its multiplication and spread to the intensity of human activity and the in-disciplined behaviour of the affected people.*

Lockdowns are no sure cure or antidote against the dreaded virus; they have only limited utility of temporarily slowing down spread of infection since the process is directly proportional to the intensity of human interaction, especially in closed and congested spaces.

Lockdowns frustrate people because human-beings are social animals; they like to meet, talk, and celebrate—and they hate restrictions, especially when the same are long and repetitive in nature. Fatigue of lockdowns is a well-known phenomenon with several undesirable effects on physical, as well as mental wellbeing of affected people.

> *Some experts felt that it would be wiser to allow the virus a free run while protecting only the vulnerable sections of society and let the herd immunity develop in subject populations to allow self-limiting of the virus when not enough unexposed people are left for it to jump from one to another with the resultant natural distancing.*

Only Sweden experimented with the free-run approach and the damages to society caused by the dreaded pandemic weren't more serious than those suffered by several other countries which relied on inconvenient lockdowns.

When restrictions are eased, or lifted entirely, people tend to hurry up for getting back on lost time and gain normality. There is a tendency amongst people to cluster on beaches and in bars, restaurants, and gyms etc. And Corona loves this human frailty and jumps from one person to another, multiplying with gusto and creating a stream of victims. It's a win-win situation for the cunning virus.

> *Hence, when there are restrictions or lockdowns, first the pathogen retreats temporarily and with the opening up or un-locking, its multiplication gains pace corresponding to human activity's intensity causing chain reactions of multiplication and infections, resulting into rush to hospitals and un-nerving/ confusing authorities who tend to make more mistakes and help the virus take revenge on the just freed society.*

These accelerating infections are termed as a 'wave', second or third, depending upon location specificities. These waves are more of a rule than exception; given human social behaviour frailties (as they exist presently) that are bound to cause such situations—and more frustration and confusion is a consequence. Governments, mostly scientifically poor formations of politicians and administrative machinery, have no other tool at their disposal. Only a handful of such formations were able to work intelligently and get on the pathogen more successfully. Small nations, especially those either led by technologists, or where political formations paid adequate attention to expert advice, did well in fight against the great Corona.

Second wave or surge, however, occurred as a rule; only severity and duration of the episode varied. In USA, India and Brazil, all of which had autocratic governance suffered the highest damages. First spread of the pandemic and second wave in these cases were seen merged with each other, without any gap or space between the two. To an extent, even in UK the virus was seen exhibiting the same type of behaviour. In contrast, Spain, France, Germany, Belgium, Russia and some other countries were seen having clear gaps between the first spread and subsequent wave or waves of the dreaded virus.

Early October, Spain's capital went under lockdown and the people so affected were unhappy. Similarly, France reported over 20,000 daily count of new cases and had to put its four major urban centres under restrictions while its hospitality sector complained loudly.

And by middle of October 2020, UK was forced to implement three tier restrictions on mobility of people and operations of hospitality outlets. The situation, as dictated by the dreaded pandemic, was truly oppressive as the whole EU region was put on a mat by the so-called second wave in October/November 2020. Some countries went through third wave too.

* * *

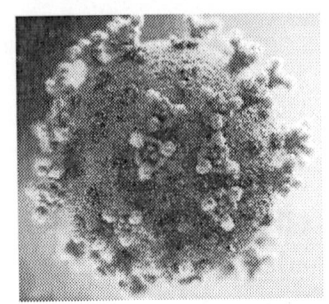

EPISODE 26

KHAKI BRUTALITY IN CORONA TIMES

The Corona period of 2020 was characterised with lockdowns almost all over the world. The job of implementing restrictions on movement of people for commerce or otherwise were vested with police and other paramilitary forces. It was seen that the behaviour of these law enforcing agents differed a great deal in developed countries, on one hand and in the developing world of Asia, Africa, and South Americas, on the other. In Asia too police were polite and efficient in countries such as Japan, South Korea, Taiwan, New Zealand, and Singapore. But in countries like India, Pakistan, and several others the story was different.

> *Here, the police were seen wielding stick and hurling abuses while pushing people off the road even when they were out for procuring essential items of day to day use and/or attending to medical emergencies. Indian police was particularly stick happy even when unemployed and homeless citizens walked long distances to their homes in rural areas; hungry, thirsty and tired they faced police brutality as if they were under instructions from higher authorities.*

In small towns and even in metros people who ventured on two-wheeler or bicycles to pick up milk for children and/or medicines for sick were showered with a heartless hail of sticks. No compassion was shown as if the perpetrators were wholly devoid of emotions.

> *People were threshed even when they fell on the road. Daily wagers' carts of vegetables and fruits were overturned, and a shower of sticks was the reward for the poor people. Some police officers were seen crushing the so spilled fruits and vegetables with their jeeps and motorbikes.*

Several TV channels presented these scenes of senseless brutality—and no one from the administration that controlled these brutal, so-called law enforcing forces, bothered to intervene. These Khaki clad brutal agents of the anti-people state proved that they were totally untrained, except in use of sticks and showering of abuses on poor and weak. There was an obvious bias against the poor; those who moved in swanky cars were spared of this senseless brutality.

In Pakistan, police were seen treating doctors and other paramedics, who had taken to road as to protest against non-availability of PPEs in hospitals, with brutal shower of sticks, kicks and abuses. This kind of behaviour wasn't seen anywhere in the countries of developed world.

> *In USA, the heavily armed and racist white police was seen killing unarmed African Americans as if they were wild animals licensed for culling. Killing of George Floyd sparked worldwide protests that lasted over three months. There was intense demand for substantial reformation of the police force, on one hand and defunding and de-arming of the racist police, on the other.*

In South American countries too, a tendency towards police brutality against poor people stressed by the dreaded pandemic, was visible to a considerable extent. Inefficient and autocratic governments loved controls and their police relished the same to an unlimited extent.

* * *

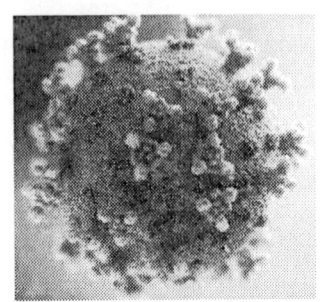

EPISODE 27

LASTING SCARS OF CORONA ON THE SOCIETY

Corona didn't only kill people—it left several lasting scars on mental and physical structure of the society. Thousands of people died lonely death, without their loved ones being around them.

Relatives also couldn't give proper burials and/or funerals to loved ones who fell to the dreaded Corona. These and related factors negatively affected human thought process leading to:

1. Those who survived the Corona attack and the ones who lost their loved ones to the deadly pandemic were seen accumulating a massive load of uncomfortable feelings—gilt and remorse for those who couldn't attend to loved ones—and the surviving ones for fear of lingering after-effects not disappearing fast enough. Not being able to properly attend to their departing relatives was, indeed, a great moral and emotional load, on one hand and failing in their religious rituals, on the other, created a lingering doubt in regard to peaceful movement of the departed souls. It created a lasting stress in the post-pandemic society.

2. Those who tested positive and were forced into isolation at

home or in detention centres too suffered a deep psychological scar on account of fear of death encountered for weeks so spent in lonely environment. *And the ones who reached hospitals and survived the dreaded ailment after long struggle in congested environment of death and despair had their thought process deeply dented.*

The cumulative impact of the stressful development substantially increased incidence of mental ailments in the society. Depression turned into an infectious ailment in the post-Corona society and several well-organised hospitals established post-recovery consultation centres for dealing with the lingering physical and non-physical complications. Attendance at psychologists' and other mental health experts' clinics increased disproportionately. The incidence of suicides increased a great deal in several societies.

3. As a consequence of this situation, visits to churches and temples by the surviving persons and/or their relatives increased significantly; the fear of unknown had grabbed them in a strange grip. And, on the reverse, in some cases people lost faith in their traditional religions and turned non-believers. *Their prayers, when faced with the dreaded disease, had not worked; they concluded that if God existed, then in such demanding situations it failed to do his job properly.* He had no business of abandoning them and their loved ones to the vicious ravages of the dreaded Corona.

4. In general, *the happiness quotient of the people, almost world over, seemed to have decreased a great deal—and superstition took deeper roots in the society. More people, especially the aged with disposable means, turned to charity in an increased manner.*

As a result of increased superstition and dented psychology of the masses, business of astrologers, pundits and fortune-tellers in the society gained a great deal. Some Indian astrologers even went ahead to claim that the Corona pandemic was a product of adverse planetary combinations where Rahu, Ketu and Sanni played vicious games on people.

5. *Human society seemed to have reached new normal in almost all aspects of life and its interactions in the post-pandemic period, with its altered thought lines of faith, behaviour, and practices.* People's method of greeting each other too was now a great deal different. Speaking through masks, keeping distance at work as well as pleasure became a new normal. Welcoming customers with masks on and hence with hindered smile was neither normal nor welcome in-service sector in any manner.

6. Tourism and hospitality industry took a long time to come out of the Covid-19 dictated downturn—and it wasn't clear as when was it to reach the pre-2020 level; probably not for several years—and several of its component businesses were destined to fold-up. In the process, businesses related to the travel and entertainment industry, especially the small and standalone ones, closed un-ceremoniously.

7. Unemployment lingered for long at unsustainably elevated levels never known in the past—making poor and vulnerable suffer a great deal. Lines grew longer on charity run soup kitchens and free food distribution centres.

8. A section of people, particularly those who recovered from the disease and, to an extent, the doctors and care givers were stigmatized for its lingering effect. In backward countries police took long time to understand its original duties as they had gone fond of wielding the stick while enforcing long lockdowns.

9. *Many governments, some even the democratically elected ones, became accustomed to autocratic and/or dictatorial methods to which they had resorted to unhindered during the pandemic period.* The unhindered power tasted by them

was difficult to give up. And numerous welfare-oriented schemes which earlier were run to benefit the poor were dropped or curtailed substantially.

Post-corona societies came under greater assault of tax-collectors as several governments' treasuries had gone empty during the Covid-19 run.

10. *Globalisation suffered an unsung partial demise as governments, based on their struggle to procure essential items during the pandemic, turned to greater localisation and/or self-reliance. Trust in Chinese goods, in general, suffered a decline.*

11. International cooperation and functioning of UN based organisations suffered due to political struggle for supremacy between USA, the old superpower, on one hand and China, the emerging one, on the other. International aid for developmental works too suffered a setback on account of reduced availability of funds. Countries in Africa with accumulated Chinese debts struggled with rescheduling or repayments. There were many other unexpected setbacks to international interactions.

12. More economic migrants from sub-Saharan tract in Africa moved to north with the hope of eventual crossing over to Europe.

13. *Dictators got an unearned lease of life as in the corona-affected society's opposition political parties weakened a great deal. Several democratically elected governments developed autocratic tendencies as they found it inconvenient to give up powers assumed in the pandemic stressed period.*

14. Universities in Europe, USA, Canada, and Australia now offered lower aids to foreign students. Job opportunities too for new graduates and IT personnel seemed reduced. Trump's *'America First'* emphasis in USA lingered on.

Schools and colleges, with the need for physical distancing and sanitization attempted to unexpectedly greater reliance on digital and virtual methodologies and practices.

15. Struggling oil prices and resultant low incomes affected armament trade too, but intra-state and interstate struggles continued unabated.

In brief, no aspect of human life remained in the pre-pandemic state. Everything altered in a varying manner—creating situations of new normal in every aspect of human life.

* * *

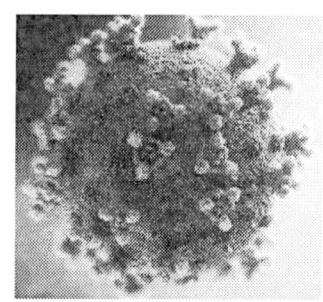

EPISODE 28

LIFTING LOCKDOWNS AND EASING OF RESTRICTIONS

Lockdowns, in the first place, were complex decisions to arrive at and difficult to implement. *In case of some countries where politics and science didn't conflict, lockdown decisions were timely and had good impact towards limiting damage to human life by the dreaded Covid-19.* In case of Italy, Spain, France, UK, and USA which suffered the largest damage to human life, these decisions were delayed—and were not wholly smooth. It happened primarily on account of difference of opinion as what to do and when to impose restrictions on human mobility and social contacts.

> *Sweden was, in fact, the only country not to impose lockdown since the authorities there felt that the critical requirement for slow movement of the virus was social or physical distancing and a disciplined people could do that without going through too harsh measures. They kept schools, colleges, restaurants, and malls open and commercial life moved normally all through March, April and May when rest of the world went under varied periods of lockouts.*

The medical authorities, including virologists, there thought that there was no point in restricting movement of the pathogen in the human society. For effective results a population must achieve a herd immunity (about 60% or so people should contact the disease) for the purpose. In any case, some loss of human life was inevitable when such a pandemic struck. A lockout only temporarily disrupted virus's spread while it delivered disruptive blow to economy. This approach continued all through the pandemic year 2020.

After six to seven weeks of lockdown, almost all countries that had so suffered, felt an urgent need for some free movement and opening places of work and commerce was seen turning into a compulsion. For most nations to arrive at a decision to open up was, in fact, more difficult than what it was while imposing the same. While deciding to impose the lockdown they had felt powerful and decisive but in case of the opening up decision fear of second wave of infections weighed heavily in mind of most governments. But the need for fresh air and some exercise for people who were holed up for weeks—and also the necessity for freeing industry and businesses from limitations of lockouts had become urgent.

For President Trump, rescuing US businesses and industry from limitations of the lockout, had become most urgent considering his personal and political need for winning election in November 2020.

Almost everywhere, opening up of small businesses and retail points was seen being urgent for their survival. Human society's capacity to remain in lockout was indeed limited. It damaged purse as well as minds of people and wasn't sustainable in the long run.

Some countries like Spain started with opening up construction industry on priority where physical distance maintenance was seen technically feasible. Others opted for imposing employees' attendance limitations and prescribed measures for avoiding customers crowding on counters or in any closed space. In some country's restaurants were allowed only to operate takeaway services. For some countries opening of hair dressing and other small joints was seen essential for the wellbeing of the stressed society.

And most of the countries said that in case the infection rebounded then the lockdown restrictions could be re-imposed on selective basis.

> *Without exception, all countries of the world were seen struggling with the process of lifting of lockdown restrictions because behaviour of the virus in so eased situations was uncertain. Opening up was a risky operation and needed caution as well as planning for corrective measures if need arose. Several countries did suffer resurgences but, in most cases, except USA and Europe, such outbreaks were managed with sustained efforts.*

India exhibited massive incompetence and insensitivity in its decisions regarding lockdown timing and its durations. The lockdown that it had hurriedly imposed on 24th March 2020, was extended three times in the months of April, and May creating hugely inhuman conditions for migrant labour, on one hand and over 400 million of people where families struggled in one room dwellings, some with three generations crowding together, on the other, it was a huge nightmare. The so-called need for observing physical distancing was a wholly infeasible idea in countries like India, Bangladesh, Nigeria etc where a huge majority of population lived in one room dwellings.

In USA, President Trump's compulsion for a quick opening up of businesses and industry created huge controversies between his administration, on one hand and with state governors, on the other. During a Congressional hearing in mid-May, 2020, it caused nation's top heath scientists and medical experts to resort to warnings that too much of a hurry towards opening up of businesses and industries could cost the country dearly in terms of loss of human life.

In United Kingdom Prime Minister, Boris Johnson, advised people to *'stay alert'* if going out for work was unavoidable and even in parks and gardens maintenance of physical distancing was made necessary. Restaurants commenced with takeaway services. Denmark and some other countries opened schools with prescribed restrictions on occupancy and inter-child spacing.

> *One country in Europe even experimented with a robotic dog to go around and help maintain physical distancing in parks and gardens.*

There was no uniformity of approach in the opening up process amongst countries except that all were worried and observed caution.

The struggle to open businesses and places of collective interactions saw nightmarish situations as the dreaded pandemic's passage moved beyond middle of the year 2020. The chaos continued unabated all through the pandemic year 2020 and into 2021.

* * *

EPISODE 29

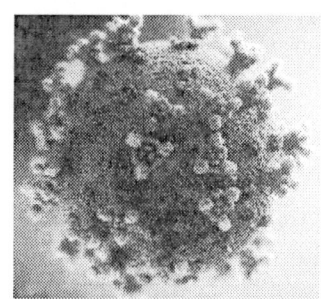

LONG-TERM IMPACT OF CORONA ON HUMAN SOCIETY

Coronavirus is a long hauler bio-agent. It is not in a hurry to do its job and disappear for good. It seems that Corona loves the in-disciplined environment of the human society i.e., its follies related to collective enjoyment in congested and closed spaces—its sense of liberty and desire to deviate from rules and regulations suggested (not harshly imposed) by experts and authorities.

Hence, Corona shall live with us for long, multiplying, surging, and resurging at will, until and unless the human society collectively amended its ways. And that change will not come early and easily.

In light of the above, people will have to learn to live with the virus, making mistakes and being punished. Corona is not a forgiver; it has no element of compassion and/or oversight. It is a biological energy that follows certain basic rules. And it wouldn't be easy for human beings to live with this invisible enemy. They will suffer and grieve. In the process all human activities, economic and otherwise, shall suffer, prominent of which are briefly described herein.

Globalisation, the elements of which carried the dreaded Corona world over, will suffer a crippling blow. It may never recover to the pre-2019 heights.

A tendency not to be over-dependent on others, at least for critical needs, has been visible all through the Corona affected period. It will have some positive influence too, especially on lower strata of the society since increased local output of essential goods and services is bound to cause enhanced employment for those at the bottom of the pyramid.

Out of the main elements that had enabled globalisation to achieve the undesirable or unsustainable heights of pre-Covid-19 period, aviation or air travel shall suffer the most. During the coming decade, it will continue to struggle to survive and will occasionally attempt to regain lost heights and efficiencies. In the process, losses will increase and several of the aviation companies shall either fold-up or just lingering on, shedding jobs, and cutting all possible corners. Only those funded by states or with deep pockets shall do reasonably well.

Thousands of aircrafts shall be junked or left idle on tarmac and aircraft manufactures shall operate on much reduced capacities. Unsold inventories shall cripple them beyond repair, in the short term.

Economy, almost all of its components, had nose-dived in the Corona period and major parts of it may take years to recover. Some may have to just fold up, thus aggravating sufferings of a section of the society. In general, GDPs of countries, with few exceptions, may dive in the ranges of 5-10 percent. Economic depression, even deeper than that experienced in 1930s, looked to have a good possibility of emergence.

> *While Wall Street might continue to shine, people of street i.e., the common folks, shall have their troubles intensified a great deal. While returns to shareholders shall grow, the share of labour will diminish.*

Enhanced inequality and poverty shall be the most significant by-product of Covid-19 manifestations, apart from deaths and related sufferings.

Social capital, charities and compassion shall suffer a painfully long impact. Human values shall deteriorate a great deal—and selfishness and negativity in the society is bound to surge in the Covid-19 affected era.

Cultural capital of humanity that includes, amongst others, theatres, music concerts, cinema and films shall struggle for long before reaching pre-Covid-19 situation.

Sports may, however, recover more easily because of (a) the energy levels of the relatively young people involved, (b) high energy expressions of audience involved, and (c) large finances and sponsors' stakes.

World food output reduction and resultant shrinkage of availability to lower sections of the society is a great possibility in the post-Covid-19 period. Famines and resultant migrations might have to be faced by the already stresses society. Malnutrition is sure to raise its uglier head in several Asian and African states.

Automation in business and industry will tend to grow when labour deficient countries attempt to go more self-reliant. For instance, Japan intends to resort to the greater use of robots in view of its aging population and reducing labour force.

From whatsoever angle one looks, the next generation waiting to join the work force during the third decade of the century, will suffer reduced opportunities of employment and hence suffer substantial negative stress related to work and livelihood. Skills mismatch will continue to complicate matters a great deal.

> *Digital divide in the human society will turn into a perplexing challenge since a large section of the population, on one hand, lacks access to internet and computers and isn't able to pay for the same, on the other.*

Health infrastructure may attract more investments in rich countries while the developing and third world countries shall continue to be incapable to face Covid-19 type emergencies any more successfully in the future. Situation in South Asia's corruption and poverty hit regions like Bihar and UP and some societies in sub-Saharan Africa may not see light at end of the tunnel for many more years.

> *Pharma industry all over the world shall earn higher returns in the post-Covid-19 environment.*

Demand for greater investments in social welfare measures will become acute but there wouldn't be matching availability of funds because of imbalance in priorities of various governments.

Human capital shall remain under stress almost all over the world for several years to come. In brief, the Covid-19 stressed human society is in for long-lasting negative living and working environment for several years to come.

> *Mental health situation is bound to deteriorate almost all over the world under load of lingering grief for loss of near and dears, on one hand, and reduced incomes, on the other.*

Education, private or public suffered long lasting adverse impact on account of some institutions' inability to sustain, on one hand, and difficulties in adjustment to greater emphasis on the on-line orientation, on the other.

To summarise, one can safely conclude that no part of human life, collective or individual—and business or non-business related, shall remain unaffected by the lingering adverse impact or the curse of the dreaded Corona.

> *Some experts predicted that world economy might take over a decade to recover to the pre-Covid-19 level. One of them asserted that generations of mankind might continue to suffer lingering after-effects of the Covid-19 pandemic.*

Corona is a work in progress and hence it is almost impossible to assess and/or predict its true and total negative impact on the human society.

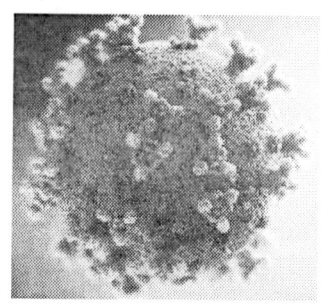

EPISODE 30

MANY BATTLES IN THE LONG CORONA WAR

Corona is an invisible and treacherous enemy. Additionally, being a brand-new pathogen nothing much was known about it. Its origin too was shrouded in mystery. For these reasons there wasn't any known treatment or vaccine available against it and hence humanity has indeed been at a loss as how to deal with it.

Within three months of its appearance in Wuhan city of China, it had raced to cover the whole world, except the icy contingent around the South Pole. When not handled carefully, it exhibited capability to destroy large stretches of humanity with the speed of wildfire. Bergamo in northern Italy and New York, the world's financial capital, suffered maximum wrath of the dreaded enemy, infecting a large chunk of the population, and killing significant number of residents. In latter part of the Covid year 2020, it created great chaos in USA, Brazil, India, and the EU region.

The way Corona turned into a world-wide tsunami in one go and punishing most the ignorant and careless, the war against it turned out to be a long, messy and a costly one. In numerous countries, it initiated innumerable battles, winning most, and losing some. Coronavirus, through its great skills of appearance and spread proved that it was an expert guerrilla fighter. It appeared, attacked, and killed at expected as well as unexpected places totally at will. When will it retreat and reappear was most difficult to assess and/or predict? All known weapons available with the mankind, nuclear and/or otherwise, seemed ineffective against it. It retreated and re-attacked or surged as a skilful guerrilla force.

> *Battles against the Corona were indeed messy; the worst ones were fought in Wuhan, Bergamo, Iran, Madrid, Barcelona, London, New-York, Moscow, California, Mumbai, Delhi, and numerous other places.*

The worst war scenes were seen in hospitals where people died like flies. Morgues ran out of space for dead and, in many cases, dead bodies were seen stored in refrigerated trucks. In countries like Spain ice rinks were acquired for storage of the dead. Burial rituals were given a go-by at most places. Churches weren't allowed to conduct funeral services. At some burial grounds, especially in backward countries, people were agitated not to let the dead be buried on account of fear for the spread of the disease in neighbourhoods. Huge burial grounds in Brazil with freshly dug graves in long rows presented a dreadful scenario. Coffin makers worked overtime yet couldn't meet the demand—at several places dead bodies were just rolled into mass graves.

> *Remains of war against Corona were seen scattered in streets and lanes of affected cities and towns.*

Shops, restaurants, bars were locked up and nothing moved, except stray dogs. Iconic squares and plazas were deserted. Parks were fully devoid of visitors and iconic avenues like Champs-Élysées in Paris were starved of walkers and visitors.

In some small and backward towns, dead bodies were left unattended for days. And at many places wooden burial boxes went out of supply forcing usage of cardboard boxes or mere plastic bags were employed for the purpose of disposing of the dead.

When battles subsided, normalcy took months—and in some cases, it took years for the situation to return to some normalcy. In fact, the human society never regained the pre-Corona social norms and behaviour for a long time.

> *And the dreaded enemy was never open to negotiations for final settlement. Possibly, it hated soap and water—and other sanitation measures.*

Its supply and regrouping systems are amazingly efficient—and hence it could fight long and frustrating battles with amazing success.

Covid-19 demonstrated that it is a long duration fighter and hence its battles extended far beyond the year 2020.

* * *

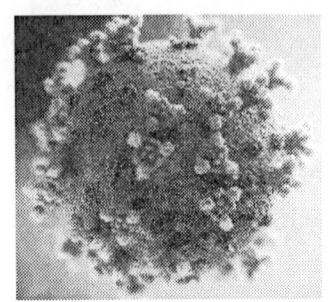

EPISODE 31

MASTER OF RESURGENCE AND LOCKDOWN GAMES

Covid-19 is not a simple pathogen that would infect and eventually disappear for good. It lies low and persists on human frailties, regroups and attacks mercilessly as opportunity arises. Being intelligent, it knew full well that human-beings were bound to return to their old habits and, being social in nature, they will congregate in congested environments, thus making the cunning Covid-19's job easier i.e., to jump from one person to another and reproduce at break-neck speed to infect and cause a surge.

> *Human beings, not knowing the deceitful enemy well enough, tended to panic and saw lockdown as the only means to limit or restrict the virus's multiplication.*

Lockdown is not a cure; it only puts some roadblocks in path of the dreaded pathogen. While it temporarily restricts the virus's spread, economy takes a downward spin and society is put in a catch-22 situation.

After a few weeks' lockdown human-beings cautiously ease restrictions and start mingling in their livelihood and/or entertainment environment presuming that the invisible enemy had been humbled but such assumptions normally remain far from being true. The dreadful virus keeps multiplying in human bodies asymptomatically and as soon as its numbers are large enough again for a fight, it strikes back, surprising the populace and governance authorities with punishing resurgence. Panic again takes over the apparatuses of governance—and the frequent response normally is to again lock-up the already suffering people. The virus loves the so emerging situations, and it is back with a vengeance in the game of attack, retreating and regrouping—causing the dangerous game of surge (or resurge) and lockdown (or re-lockdown) ruining both the human society as well as its economy (livelihood) in its dangerous game against the mankind.

> *All over the world, country after county, have fallen into the trap of the deadly virus, except one or two that didn't resort to lockdown and allowed the virus run a lonely normal course.*

Beginning with the Asian region where the dreadful virus had initially exposed its fangs, countries like China, Japan, South Korea, New Zealand, Australia, and Singapore, amongst others, resorted to lockdowns of differing durations and severity. And they suffered resurgences of varying intensity within weeks of lifting of painful lockdowns—and economies suffered job losses and GDP growth fall.

In South Asia, except Sri Lanka and Bhutan, countries suffered cycles of lockdowns and resurgences—and economies were ruined significantly. In desperation, authorities in Iran with its crippled economy and a strong flow of resurgence in early July 2020 announced that its economy couldn't bear another lockdown and allowed the virus to take its own course. It was possibly a wise move.

> *India's case was that of an organised confusion. After the 24 March national wide lockdown which was extended four times without a clear objectivity, lack of clarity in approach was seen missing. Here,*

> *the Central Government had proclaimed that the Covid-19 would be humbled in just 18 days on lines of the epic battle of Kurukshetra where forces of good and righteousness had defeated massively organised evil formations some five millennia ago.*

Blinded by ignorance and arrogance, it didn't do its best to upgrade medical facilities and arrange of necessary tools such as PPE kits and ventilators. It persisted with political manipulations to (a) discredit opposition rules states and (b) bring down democratically established governments.

Covid-19, being an intelligent pathogen, went slow during extended lockdowns and, as soon as, the biological force reached critical levels of multiplication, it raised dreadful fangs in Mumbai, Dharavi, Ahmedabad, Delhi, Bengaluru, and Chennai—and also took a ride with migrant workers to rural India. Indian economy that was hugely crippled during the period didn't respond to restrictive opening-up in May and June 2020 despite greatly advertised but impractical incentives. The confused central government resorted to numerous lockdowns in the so-called containment (red and yellow) zones. Its confusion was profusely visible in its unjust scaling up of petrol and diesel retail prices that further delayed economic recovery. Covid-19 loved these confused mini-lockdowns and their hurried lifting. It enjoyed the game of hide and seek while the authorities, more often than not, made numerous mistakes.

> *Central Asia, being less connected and sparsely populated escaped punishing beatings at hands of the dreaded virus. Further, West-Asia, except the Jewish state, too avoided massive losses at hands of the Covid-19, possibly because most of the communities there were free of beaches, bars, spas and other related closely interacting components of the culture.*

Additionally, Saudi Arabia had promptly closed down the Islamic tourism centres of Macca and Madina, thus denying Covid-19 an easy ride with pilgrims.

Europe which suffered the greatest knocks of the dreadful virus all through March, April, and May—and then August onwards for a long period. Countries such as Italy, Spain, France, and UK were devastated in terms of loss of human life also suffered lasting damages to their economies. They were seen in a hurry to open up crippled economies in months of May and June since all of them wanted to salvage summer tourism incomes and job revivals. Germany and countries of the northern region had escaped with relatively minor damages. Germany, Spain, Belgium, Portugal, and some others suffered resurgences and relock-downs in June and July while others feared the same fate as summer advanced.

Maximum hurry to open up the devastated economy was seen in USA and its constituent states suffered massive resurgences in June and July that was never seen diminishing all through the year—extending well into the year 2021. President Trump was unwisely coxing infection suffering states to open up economies in light of his re-election priorities. He even instigated his supporters to agitate for the same. In July Florida, Arizona, Texas, and California suffered such crippling surges that figures of daily infections reached all time peaks. Experts and scientists warned of dire consequences. There was great rush for hospital admissions and Covid-19 gleefully enjoyed its supremacy in the world's most advanced societies. Reluctantly, President Trump was seen adorning a face mask when he visited an armed forces' medical facility. And it was by now evident that the unpredictable President had lost his re-election chances on account of his conflicting statements and interactions. Despite the grim state of Covid-19 related situations in the whole country he was persistently campaigning for opening up of schools and other educational institutions. He even threatened millions of foreign students studying in American universities to cancel their visas and deport them if their studies continued solely in virtual mode. Education experts differed a great deal with his fulminations.

> *And Covid-19 was seen greatly enjoying its massive success in putting a Superpower to mat and pinning it down mercilessly.*

Further down south, Brazil received the second worst drubbings at hands of Covid-19 as its President consistently conflicted with states and actively opposed lockdowns. Corona took best advantage of the governance conflict and ruined the Brazilian society as well its economy in a manner that for decades after-effects of the chaos were sure to be suffered by the largest South American country.

Several other countries in the region too suffered devastating impact of lockdowns and opening up confusion and compulsions imposed by the mighty virus. Its masterly strategy of pinning the mankind to ground and causing massive losses of life and livelihood was seen winning hands down.

* * *

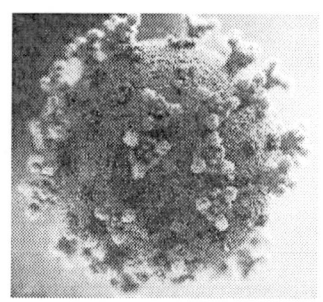

EPISODE 32

MEDICAL FRATERNITY FACED A SITUATION OF NO SURE CURE

Coronavirus had put the world medical community in real quandary. The virus was new, and doctors didn't know how to treat patients infected by it. Its symptoms largely confused the situation to seasonal flu, but most flu medications didn't work.

> *The medical fraternity was left to jugad i.e., treating the corona cases symptomatically administering paracetamol for controlling fever and treating respiratory distress with oxygen and ventilators.*

The latter, including the PPEs, were often in short supply and in many cases doctors and nurses had to risk their own lives. Many protested but administrations often were unsympathetic to such complaints.

Some doctors tried hydroxyl chloroquine, a malaria drug as a preventive for the frontline workers for some unconfirmed benefits.

Several countries asked India for supply of the antipyretics as well as the HCQ. President Trump of USA at one stage even threatened India for consequences if it blocked supply of the drugs in question to USA that had come under severe attack of the dreaded

Corona by the first week of April 2020.

> *Several medical centres and hospitals experimented with extracting serum from patients who had gotten well after infection and had developed anti-bodies in their blood (and were willing to donate the same for the benefit of critically ill patients).*

The only reliable hope for relief was development of vaccines which still looked months away, if not years. But scientist's world over were trying hard and the medical community just had to wait patiently for the vaccine-year 2021.

> *In the New Year, despite arrival of several vaccines the great virus decided to mutate furiously and was ready for more serious battles with the already exhausted medical fraternity.*

The second wave in India (April/May 2021) had put doctors into a really tough situation when in face of severe shortage of oxygen, they often had to make choice as which patient to save and which ones let fade away. Further, they came under great stress when the disease took an unprecedentedly large toll of patients due to one or the other reason—or when they couldn't save even their own friends and relatives. Last minute encounter with dying patients when none of their relatives came forward to hold hands and say parting words was indeed most challenging. Disclosing news of death to relatives was again a greatly stressful moment—and massive stress accumulation in such difficult working situations for long hours took not only an emotional toll of doctors and nurses but a large number of they themselves fell to the dreaded virus and/or ended up infecting their own family members. Unsympathetic attitude of governments and long delays in payment of salaries further added to the misery of these frontline worriers.

* * *

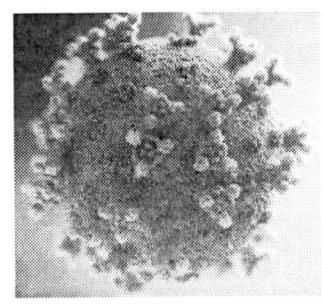

EPISODE 33

POLITICS OF CORONAVIRUS SPREAD AND CONTAINMENT

Did Corona limit itself to killing some vulnerable people? Not really! It adversely affected almost all aspects of human life. Without going into details, it can safely be said that politics, international as well as domestic, suffered a great deal at hands of the pandemic—because the dreaded disease affected human thought process and caused stress and uncertainties. Since politics is a product of thought interactions in collective environment, the great pandemic adversely impacted international as well as domestic political interactions—some of which were short-lived in nature while others were seen lingering on for a long time.

Most prominently, the pandemic caused distrust between USA and China; the former actively accused the latter of wilfully spreading the deadly pathogen world over –or at least it (a) did not rigorously attempt to limit the pathogen and control it right in Wuhan, its place of origin, (b) didn't warn the world timely, and (c) colluded with the WHO to initially cover up the episode. The US President consistently grew critical of Chinese behaviour and called it even a *'dragon's conspiracy'* to damage the world economy as well as the social order of the pre-2019 world community. How would the post-pandemic world situation benefit the red dragon wasn't clarified but the red objectivity seemed substantially clear. The Chinese government vehemently denied the US President's accusation, but the issue intensified as the presidential election in US neared. And it persisted well into years that followed.

Thus, the pandemic caused active distrust between the world Superpower and the dragon's growing economic as well as military clout—and it dragged many other nations into the emerging controversy. This growing distrust of the dragon and its objectivity amongst pro-Western counties like Australia, Taiwan, Japan, and numerous others seemed to cause an uncomfortable unease in an increasing manner.

> *Within USA no opposition politician from the Democratic party or otherwise supported the President Trump's line except that general distrust of China, in a major section of the world community, seemed growing up as the Covid year 2020 gave way to 2021. And when in power after election democrats too actively dived into the lasting controversy.*

During the pandemic period several countries imported PPEs and testing kits from China but most of them doubted the quality and reliability of the same. India had imported five million test kits in the months of March-April 2020 and the whole consignment turned out to be substandard and gave misguiding results. Since the supplier didn't admit the mistake the whole consignment had to be sent back and the episode seemed to add to the pre-existing mistrust towards Chinese supplies and its commercial practices.

The substandard or non-functioning Chinese testing kits even caused some friction between Indian medical authorities like ICMR and health ministry, on one hand and several state governments, on the other since they had to use the same during the active pandemic crisis.

> *As a consequence of the pandemic that killed hundreds of thousand people around the world and crippled the world economy, trust between the WHO (which was supposed to offer guidance and support in such critical situations) and several suffering states declined considerably. President Trump even suspended US financial support to this international organisation.*

In European Union (EU) distrust grew between the southern states—namely Italy, Spain and France which suffered most on account of the dreaded pandemic, on one hand and the richer states of northern Europe, on the other. In fact, at one point, majority of Italian citizens were reported doubting the utility of their country remaining a part of the EU. None of the EU members, in fact, came to the rescue of Italian government when it was pushed to the ground by the deadly virus. In democracies where multi-party system operated, interparty tensions were seen spurting as those in opposition were bound to oppose governing elements for not handling the situation well with needed effectiveness.

In general, it seemed that the pandemic had caused significant reduction in international trust and cooperation and it wasn't clear as how long this undesirable impact was to persist before disappearing fully.

* * *

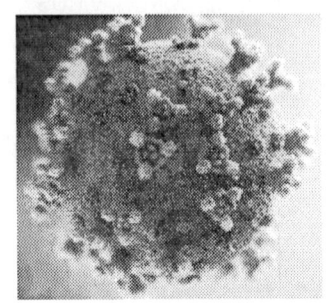

EPISODE 34

LIKELY DARK SCENARIO OF THE POST-CORONA ERA

During the Corona period most governments resorted to lockdowns and several other restrictions on movement and economic activities of masses. It is possible that as a consequence of Corona period practices most governments might develop residual taste for multilateral controls. Controls give a sense of power which some of them might find difficult to give up.

> *Distorted management of news and news channels was widely resorted to during lockdown periods. Protection and promotion of single narrative, namely what government said and wanted to promote was seen becoming a prime concern of pro—establishment forces (official as well as non-official)—and anyone from public, opposition or rights groups commenting upon the validity or invalidity of the official narrative ran the risk of being termed, or dubbed, as anti-national or spending month or even years in jail.*

Some governments employed mobile applications (or apps in brief) to trace contacts and keep track of people involved in inconvenient activities. Mobile apps in hands of control-oriented governments had dangerous potential for misusing the same for spying on individuals who differed with government approach or policies. Personal liberties or even preferences fell in danger when control loving authorities grew fond of manipulating situations to fit into their narratives. Monopolistic tendencies were seen growing dangerously putting public welfare in danger.

There existed great potential for misuse of tracking and tracing apps to get under the skin of people and gather data that might be misused for harassing people who differed with establishment.

> *For example, in India, Belarus, Russia and Hong Kong face recognition technologies were noticed being misused to identify people who didn't follow official narratives. Several such persons were later arrested and punished, some even without specifying charges and others being slapped with draconian provisions of anti-people laws.*

Killing dissent, free flow of which is deemed essential for democratic behaviour, had become easier in Covid times—and, as a consequence, many more journalists (and those who disagreed) with independent or investigative tendency were likely to be restrained and/or put behind bars.

Controls employed during lockouts and the restrictive opening-up process posed a great danger to emergence of permit and licence raj (restrictive and discriminative governance) in several countries of Asia, Africa, and Latin America.

Surging unemployment and resultant loss of incomes in the post-Corona era of nose-diving economies will compel resources starved people to lose their meagre residences for not being able to pay rents and consequently resort to pavement living.

> *The likely dire post-Corona economic situations were seen witnessing of lengthening food lines or crowds at soup kitchens, with many first timers turning in. Number of destitute people in populace of poor countries was likely to increase.*

> *In India after the disastrous second wave poverty was seen galloping beyond expectations.*

As more and more small businesses failed to survive, rentals of commercial properties in urban complexes will suffered. The post-Corona society seemed destined to see a new normal of poverty manifestations.

Post-Corona societies will face more tensions on account of the above and related uncertainties. Diseases related to stress accumulations and resultant mental imbalances shall surge unabatedly.

> *There shall be surge of migration across continents and international borders.*

Institutions for managing international order shall weaken. USA was seen likely to suffer weakening of its international role and China might not be able to gather adequate cooperation to fill the emerging gap. As a consequence, UNO, IMF, WHO etc will see weakening of their operations. How will the Joe Biden administration in USA help in minimising these scenario is to be watched with active interest.

> *Religions too suffered at hands of the Corona. It has weakened people's faith in God and in its effectiveness—yet gatherings at churches, temples and mosques did not decrease as uncertainties of life are bound to push people in this direction.*

* * *

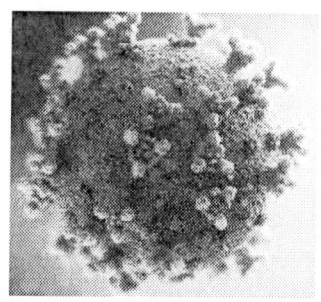

EPISODE 35

PRESIDENT TRUMP TURNED INTO A SUPER-SPREADER OF CORONA

> *In the second trimester of 2020, President Trump was pushed on to back-foot by the Biden-Harris candidacy. Despite having had an encounter with the dreaded virus he infused great energies into his re-election campaign and during the last four weeks prior to the 3rd of November vote doubled his public gatherings in key states that had potential for swinging and re-swinging at the last moment.*

His vigour seemed uncommon. For him it had turned into a do-or-die moment. He attracted good crowds and none of them cared for a mask or social distancing. All his fans and followers reflected their leader's typical contempt for the dreaded virus even though the second Corona wave was at its peak in several US states. The daily reported cases of infections crossed the level of 90,000 on end of October.

Renowned medical experts saw Trump's campaign meetings becoming *'Super-spreader'* events that were sure to enable the dreaded virus cross previous records in terms of hospitalisations and avoidable deaths. No one seemed to listen to experts and the American public, as usual, wasn't scared of the consequences. The state bureaucracy, federal or in states could do nothing, or didn't seem to be attempting to avoid a crisis situation. The opposition team of Biden and Harris that often commented upon Trump's total lack of interest, or his administration's dire failure to combat Corona, was mocked at as if it wanted to shut down the US economy in the name of fighting the virus.

> *In opinion of knowledgeable Americans, President Trump's behaviour was seen totally illogical and irresponsible—and several of them were quite vocal about it. But Trump while waging a last-ditch fight for salvaging his job didn't bother a bit. It was, indeed, so typical of the man and his personality. Some more Americans falling to the dreaded Corona wasn't his concern.*

Trump lost the election, and, in the meantime, Corona surged to create new heights of infections and loss of American lives. USA was now faced with a strong possibility of encountering a **'dark winter'** and the Christmas/New Year festival season had lost its flavour.

* * *

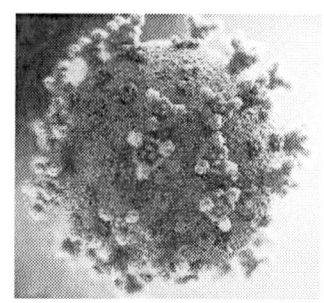

EPISODE 36

PRINCIPLES EMERGING OUT OF SPREAD OF CORONA PANDEMIC

The great pandemic's stormy spread all over the world during the first half of the year 2020 seemed to have been governed by some principles, the significant ones being:

Corona or the Covid-19 pandemic emerged in east, i.e., the Wuhan town of China. There from it moved west in a stormy manner and covered almost all the countries of the world in an unexpected manner.

> *This seemed to lead to emergence of the principle that the great pathogen moved with the movement of earth, drawing energy from this natural phenomenon of planetary movements.*

Being a fast mover, the Covid-19 during the first phase of its massive spread, preferred to ride with the high healed and fast-moving air travellers. It loved the congested and air-conditioned environment of aircrafts' interior. It could easily jump from one person to another and was then carried away thousands of miles for further action.

From the above emerged a clear principle that states:

> *The spread and intensity of the Covid-19 movement in the first phase to various countries in Europe and Asia seemed directly proportional to the number of air flights received by the respective countries from Chinese cities. London, Paris, Milano, Madrid, Frankfurt etc. received specifically a large load of the pathogen through the so moving mass of air travellers. Singapore and Moscow too were the significant recipients of the viral load in this manner. Iran and Pakistan received a good part of the viral load through ground route in addition to air travel. USA, through New York and Chicago etc. was late just by a week or so for receiving the deadly input from China. South American and African countries were the last to receive Covid-19's attention. It was the deadly virus's second but equally dangerous inning.*

During the second leg of its movement the great pathogen moved with infected individuals in automobiles and then enjoyed the congested and air-cooled environment of hotels, offices, restaurants, bars, spas, and gyms etc. This peculiar behaviour of the great virus led to emergence of another principle that stated:

> *'The Covid-19 pandemic needed close human interacting environment for jumping from one victim to another.'*

When the above became clear to medical experts, they suggested the need for human beings to observe six feet or two metre physical distancing in order to avoid and/or minimise spread of the dreaded disease. Often called social distancing, it became the major weapon in human-being's hands to fight against the dreaded virus.

The way Covid-19 pandemic smothered the whole world just within 4-5 months of its emergence in Wuhan in December 2019.

> *It led to emergence of another conclusion that the dreaded virus was non-discriminative in its dealings. It didn't differentiate in its intensity of attack based on size of the country and the nature of its governance i.e. whether democratic and/or autocratic.*

An intense study of various victim countries' infection and death data revealed that:

> *The great killer virus preferred densely populated countries (or regions) having a poor quality or less sensitive governance where decisions weren't fast enough—or not based on advice of scientists and technocrats—and weren't implemented firmly.* It loved the countries where politicians were more publicity lovers rather than sensitive to people's woes. The great virus wasn't scared of superpowers but was seen being conscious not to spend unduly large energy in well-governed countries. *South Korea, Taiwan, Singapore, New Zealand, Vietnam, Australia, Canada amongst a few others, did a credit worthy job of fighting the dreaded virus.*

It also became apparent that the pandemic was careful in not spending too much of its vital energy in countries that were ruled by female executives. They were seen by the cunning pathogen as quick acting and more sensitive to people's needs, medical and/or otherwise.

Another observation that emerged from behaviour of the Covid-19 was that:

> *'The pathogen was a non-discriminative destroyer when it came to dealing with people who carelessly or otherwise came its way.' 'Front-line workers i.e., doctors and nurses, fresh from college or experienced ones, were treated with uniform ferocity. Those who better observed the scientific principles survived relatively successfully.'*

Rulers who were publicity loving and depended a lot on tali (clappings), thali (making noise by beating utensils), candle lightings, flower petals shower etc were threshed mercilessly. *It led to the conclusion that the great virus wasn't scared away by noise or publicity against it.*

The virus wasn't in a hurry; it could lie low and strike when it suited her. It loved living with humans, and it was entirely left to the will and intelligence of the latter how to avoid the grip of the deadly pathogen. *Summer or winter didn't make a difference. Isolated and or thinly populated communities were spared dreaded punishment.* Finally, it could be easily concluded that the Covid-19 virus lived and worked based upon some specific principles. In fact, all bio-agents followed such principles.

* * *

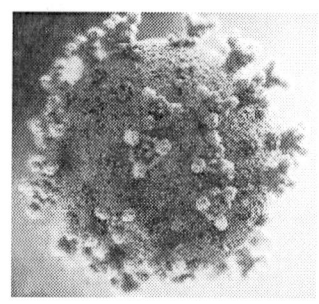

EPISODE 37

COVID-19 FIRED A RACE FOR VACCINES DEVELOPMENT

Corona is a new virus. Whether it originated from nature or was a man-made mischief became the greatest riddle of the new century. In a few months of its origin, it had overwhelmed the world as never before. Originating in November/December 2019 in Wuhan town of China, it had spread to over 200 countries of the world by end of the 1st quarter of the New-Year. It was the newest and the most dangerous pandemic faced by the mankind.

It had no known treatment or medicine that worked against the flu like symptoms that the Covid-19 caused. It was a smart pathogen that travelled (at least initially) by airways riding in and/or on bodies and clothing of tourists and businessmen. It was silent and invisible—even those initially infected by it remained asymptomatic for a week or more. It employed its silent carriers to infect other persons exponentially. Depending upon who carried it, the dreaded pathogen caused mortality in the range of 1-2 percent amongst the infected.

Senior citizens with pre-existing morbidities were its preferred prey. And it seemed to love the blacks and Hispanics in comparison to whites, yellows and/or browns. Was the virus racist in its preference? Possibly, the blacks and Hispanics came to contact it more often on account of their professions' work nature? The truth could take a long time to be verified with acceptable certainty.

By early April 2020, approximately 90 percent of the world was under dreadful lockdowns to limit its further spread. With over 1,50,000 deaths, majority of which occurred in Europe and USA, medical infrastructure of the so-called advance countries was seen cracking from all sides. There was a world-wide scramble for PPE kits and ventilators. Hundreds of doctors and paramedics had fallen to the dreaded virus while attending to the sick and dying in hospitals and nursing homes.

Medical experts and politicians often differed with each other on what approach to take against the dreaded enemy. An unprecedented human catastrophe had developed. There was almost no light at end of the ever-darkening tunnel. Since no drug or therapy worked against the horrific disease, the only face saving way-out for the scientific community of the world was to work towards finding and/or developing an effective vaccine against the dreaded enemy.

By end of April 2020 two scientific teams in USA and China—and one in UK, had claimed some progress in direction of development of a vaccine for countering the dreaded Covid-19. The UK group had even commenced initial testing trials on human volunteers. Countries like Germany, Japan and India too were in the race to developing a vaccine for the purpose. It was reported that all around the world, by middle of the year, over 150 scientific groups were active on this critical front and the WHO too extended all help and guidance in this regard.

Developing a vaccine is a complex and time-consuming process and normally, even when working at break-neck speed, it took a minimum of 12 to 18 months to succeed in this effort.

> *Production of a vaccine is one struggle—and the bigger effort involved in mass production and making the same available to everyone all over the world, without preference and/or discrimination, was a greater challenge.*

Any hurry and/or politically motivated shortcuts could be dangerous in this direction. For instance, at end of June 2020, India announced (through ICMR) that a vaccine against the dreaded virus was to be ready by 15th August of the same year. Such efforts towards half-baked and inadequately tested outputs could be dangerous for the public health. Subsequent hue and cry from several scientists, the undesirable hurry was abandoned.

Towards the second half of Covid-year 2020, it was an interesting wait by one and all. Whosoever succeeds with an effective and safe product shall earn humanity's uncontested gratitude and appreciation.

Towards middle of July 2020, the Oxford and Astra-Zeneca group announced results of its 1st phase of human trials. These were published in the Lancet medical journal and were said to be encouraging since the said vaccine not only caused anti-bodies to appear in the test individuals but also caused them to develop T-cells that imparted additional immunity. There were high expectations from this effort.

At the same time, China was reported to be testing its vaccine in Brazil and South Africa where the Covid-19 was still having a field day. India too reported initiation of human trials for its locally developed vaccine named 'Co-Vaccine'.

> *In the last week of July 2020, President Trump announced that the 3rd stage of human trials for the American vaccine 'Moderna' on over 30,000 individuals was launched as a final step towards ensuring the vaccine's availability to American public by end of the year.*

It was, indeed, a great race by the scientific community to net a vaccine as early as possible and relieve the humanity that had been pinned to ground by the tiny virus.

Russia announced in early August that its vaccine was ready for large scale applications and that the President's daughter too had taken the shoot. China went a step ahead and claimed to have granted a patient to its vaccine. In both the cases supportive data was yet to be out for independent evaluation. In first fortnight of October 2020, a vaccine expert claimed that all over the world some 321 vaccines were being worked upon and that over 190 of the same were at various stages of human trials. The whole world now waited with significant expectations for at least a handful of the vaccine development efforts to succeed and afford relief to the hugely stressed mankind.

> *Soon expectations of the hugely stressed mankind seemed being rewarded when by end of November 2020 Pfizer announced that it was ready with its product and will soon apply for needed approvals for its mass application.*

And UK hurried up to approve its emergency usage—and by end of the first week of December shipments of the vaccine were on way—to be used initially for the benefit of frontline workers and some high priority groups.

In the meantime, Moderna and Oxford-Astra-Zeneca products too had reached the finishing line and just waited for necessary approvals. Out of the three, the OAZ product seemed to offer great promise of usage in the developing world since it didn't require very low temperature facilities for its transport and application. In the meantime, Russia had commenced a large-scale vaccination drive employing its vaccine called **'Sputnik-V'**. In view of the above and related developments the year 2021 was destined to see a lot of action on the Corona vaccine front. There were six vaccines being peddled by various governments early in 2021. It was a good development for the hugely distressed mankind.

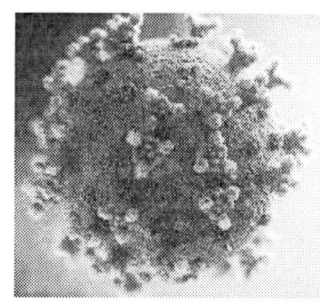

EPISODE 38

RESURGENCE: A BASIC STRENGTH OF COVID-19 VIRUS

> *Covid-19 is a highly skilled fighter. It knows when to strike and when to lie low and then re-strike again. Very much like a guerrilla force it looks for suitable opportunities to regroup and re-strike. It takes advantage of the follies and mistakes of its opponents or victims.*

And it never misjudges to strike too early or too late. Its timings are perfect and hence it had turned itself into an almost invincible killer. Covid-19 is a biological force and is endowed with inbuilt intelligence of matchless proportions. Human-beings' artificial intelligence and face recognition technologies are no match to the deadly Corona's skills.

Originating in Wuhan town of China in December 2019, it travelled world over, yet it didn't forget to resurge in Beijing a long distance away in North-East of the country, a good six months after its original emergence.

In a mild manner, it resurged in New Zealand and more severely in Australia, despite ample precautions that were taken by local authorities. Since incoming visitors weren't fully blocked, it regrouped in Victoria province of the isolated continent and caused panic. Later, towards end of June 2020, several residential blocks in Melbourne were put under lockout. Subsequently, border between the states of Victoria and New South Wales was closed in an unusual move.

> *Possibly, the virus took a ride back from the West in company of air travellers.*

Singapore had a brilliant record of dealing with the deadly virus despite being a travel and business hub—but due to some negligence it too ran into the winds of resurgence. Crowded conditions in dorms of migrant workers from Bangladesh and India, gave the intelligent virus an opportunity to strike with renewed energy of a well-rested warrior. But the city state succeeded in managing the situation exceedingly well on account of timely measures on parts of authorities.

> *It was a cakewalk for it to resurge in Iran and Pakistan where crowding in markets, on one hand and total disregard to precautions, on the other, had made the job so easier for the virus to regroup and strike.*

Some countries in Europe which were its initial victims avoided resurgence fairly well for some months, but they failed to perform adequately well against the skilful virus when travel and tourism stood reactivated at end of June 2020. The greed of authorities there, to benefit from the left-over tourist season at least partly, turned into an advantage for the deadly virus. As expected, Spain was punished by the non-forgiving Covid-19 for its extra-vigorous opening-up of tourism related travel and businesses. By middle of July 2020, Catalonia and some other parts of the country suffered Corona fires and by the 3rd week it had to again clamp down lockouts. Neighbouring France threatened closing its borders with Spain fearing that the dreaded Corona could just walk in with visitors.

RESURGENCE: A BASIC STRENGTH OF COVID-19 VIRUS

But the hugely resourceful Corona walked in through other routes and caused troublesome resurgences. And UK had imposed two weeks of compulsory quarantine on those returning from Spain and several other resurgence affected locations. Its keen desire to benefit from the left-over tourist season of the year 2020 was laid waste. *Resurging virus had confused the UK administration to the extent that it couldn't take coherent decisions all through the Corona period and by the 3rd week of September it resorted to localised lockdowns.*

Germany, a country that was relatively more successful than most others in Europe in limiting damage to its population and businesses, ran into trouble when a large meat processing factory in North-West of the country exploded with massive infection towards end of June 2020. Over 1500 of its workers were found infected and a large population of over 3,00,000 had to be quarantined. Humid and congested conditions in the large factory had provided lot of food as well as an excellent opportunity to the virus to multiply at a break-neck speed.

In UK too similar situation in meat/food processing units in Wales and Leicester led to resurgence of the deadly virus. There were some other similar cases of opportunities for the intelligent virus to rise in rebellion.

> *USA had attempted to open up its businesses and industry at a break-neck speed in May and June 2020, much against experts' advice—hence it faced a full-blown resurgence towards end of June in over 30 of its constituent states.*

It continued to devastate the country all through July. Florida, Texas, Arizona, and California did fairly badly in relation to dealing with massive resurgence towards end of June that continued full-blown through July and August 2020. Daily cases of new infection and hospital admissions had again attained or crossed the previously reached heights. In early July 2020, daily new cases in the country had crossed the 60,000 mark and the trend lasted all through July and part of August. The resurgence was significant from the point that now more young people were becoming infected. Possibly, the **'Black Lives Matter'** campaign had a hand in development of this peculiar situation. Country's hospitals were again strained to deal with the precarious situation. The whole country had gone into an unintelligent summer rush to beaches, bars, and malls. Now it suffered lockdowns of varied durations and intensities in different states. It was an apparent blow to President Trump's scheme of things and possibly to his re-election dreams in November 2020. Several of his re-election team members too were infected.

> *It seemed that the Coronavirus was more powerful than the great Superpower. It was on its knees from June through August 2020, thrashing vigorously for relief. And the country's top expert Dr Anthony Fauci had warned of serious consequences that another 1,00,000 deaths in next few months could occur if people exhibited lack of disciple—and the warning was seen almost coming true by end of August 2020.*

Europe which had showed great eagerness in June/July to open up travel and tourism related businesses in order to salvage at least part of its summer tourists' influx was in for a shock when resurgence threatened several of its constituent countries. The second wave by the deadly virus had surprised the whole EU region. Croatia suffered a dreadful surge of infection as tourists had flooded the country and in response several countries had imposed two weeks' long quarantine on their own people returning from this East European tourism location. Spain, that had shown extra eagerness to take advantage of the summer tourist season, suffered a serious backlash by the great Corona and Madrid and several other areas were again had to go under lockdown in the 2nd half of September 2020.

> *Israel, on the other hand, became the first developed country to impose a total lockdown in 2nd half of September 2020 after the tiny nation of just 9 million people suffered daily infections of over five thousand.*

RESURGENCE: A BASIC STRENGTH OF COVID-19 VIRUS

In October, Europe turned into an epicentre of Covid-19 infections. Belgium was put on a mat by the dreaded virus and authorities here feared that a tsunami of infection was on and that it wasn't capable of facing it effectively. France had put several of its urban centres including the capital under night curfew and businesses, especially hospitality sector, faced severe restrictions in terms of opening and closing times and manner of operations.

UK imposed intense restrictions and lockdown measures in a structured manner in its different regions. Ireland announced a 6-week general lockdown on 20th October. Spain continued to suffer a great deal at hands of the resurging virus and Italy too had to now resort to imposing restrictions and face masks were made mandatory for any movement out of home. Germany too continued to suffer and people in several countries protested restrictions.

Europe indeed faced most punishing surge and resurge of the dreadful virus. As a continent it seemed to have performed most miserably against the virus despite being a resourceful and technologically advanced region.

It seemed that the world should learn from the intelligent virus's skilful movements. It should be denied congested places (malls, restaurants, bars etc) and humid working environments where lack of spacing makes it easier for the virus to jump from one person to another and then multiply at will and strike at right moments.

Possibly, the mankind should also elect to go vegetarian in order to deny the virus high protein wastes to multiply furiously.

In view of the author, mankind now needed greater, more intelligent, and co-ordinated employment of science and technology, if it desired to succeed against this highly skilled enemy and avoid more punishing damages.

One could easily conclude that resurgence was more of a rule rather than an exception. Human societies, especially those led by arrogant and autocratic dispensations were sure to make mistakes and the skilful Corona was never to lose a chance to strike. Its resurgence skills are truly omnipotent.

The skilful Corona had, in-deed, put most of the governments in the world in a *'catch 22 situation'*. Economies nose-dived if lockdowns lingered on—and any hurry or carelessness in opening-ups invited punishing resurgences. No one seemed to know a fool proof way-out.

* * *

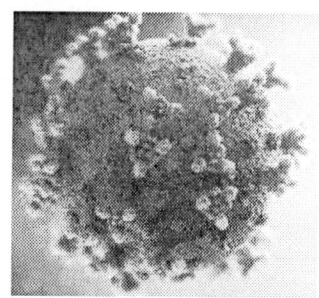

EPISODE 39

REVENUE COLLECTION PREFERRED OVER PUBLIC SAFETY

In middle of the first week of May 2020, right on commencement of the lockdown 3.0 in India, several governments (Central as well as state ones) scrambled to open liqueur shops without worrying about social distancing and public safety. In Delhi, Chennai, Mumbai and several other cities and towns, miles long lines of customers wanting to purchase wine and other alcoholic brews were seen hours before opening time of state owned or licensed shops. When shops opened, the crowd surged towards counters and police had to struggle to keep people in some minimum order—and, in several cases, the liqueur shops closed down within hours because of police's inability to keep surging customers under control.

> Seeing a great opportunity for collection of large revenues, governments jumped to raise taxes in rage of 70-100 percent and when liqueur vends opened next day customers were seen surging again to pick up drinks of their choice or whatsoever was available. Stocks flew away unexpectedly fast, perhaps because over 40 days lockdown of the large populace had stressed the people to limits of tolerance. They wanted some escape from the imposed misery.

> *During the lockout they had nothing to be engaged with except listening to noisy TV channels that sang only repetitive government propaganda, which was either rich in falsehood or attempted polarization of the masses on lines suited to the administration. Public, perhaps, had seen an opportunity for escape from the stress that had accumulated in over 6 weeks' time.*

Unmindful of the miseries of migrant workers who had taken to roads in large numbers (hungry, thirsty and sick) to reach their homes thousands of miles away when several state governments had conspired to deny them bus and/or train transport for the purpose, in the most inhuman and undemocratic way. There wasn't any social or physical distancing involved while the migrant labour on roads struggled against multiple state-imposed miseries.

Similarly, the long lines of customers waiting outside liqueur shops hours before scheduled opening didn't bother various state administrations about the need for the so-called social distancing because revenue collection compulsions overrode the need for minimising spread of the dangerous Covid-19 pandemic.

> *The revenue loving governments in India (states as well as the Central one) made piles of money when world crude prices were at historic low in March and April 2020—but their revenue hunger seemed insatiable.*

Hence, they raised taxes on retail of petrol and diesel to historic highs—consequently pushing inflation in an unprecedented manner. They didn't worry about the inflation dried public in India—or the poor and middle class didn't really exist for them. Welfare of public wasn't the governments' concern—just publicity about the same was enough for desensitising the people and to achieve their stated and/ or unstated anti-people objectivity. In such situations, the difference between a democracy and dictatorship vis-à-vis people's welfare seemed to disappear entirely.

India wasn't alone in states' attempts to pursue anti-people policies where they preferred revenue collection through hurried up opening up of businesses and industry.

> *USA was the most prominent case where President Trump consistently called for opening up of states for business all through May, June and July 2020—and, as a result, the struggling Superpower suffered a massive surge of Corona infections and resultant high hospital admissions and deaths right in June and July months.*

Trump's mishandling of the Covid-19 situations, the hurry towards opening up of businesses and industry, despite high rates of infections, amongst others, later on threatened to cost him his presidency.

Brazil's case was like that of the USA where President Jair Bolsonaro had consistently conflicted with state governors in his attempts to unlock businesses despite massive rampage of the Covid-19 in the country. But the personal cost in his case was much smaller than that suffered by Trump.

There were several other cases, but of much smaller magnitude, where states had made hurry to earn revenues by too early lifting of restrictions on businesses, especially those related to travel and tourism—and consequently suffered surges and resurges of the deadly virus.

> *The struggle of state establishments to find a balance between saving lives and livelihood continued well beyond the end of the Covid year 2020 and 2021.*

* * *

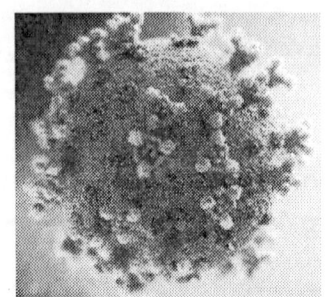

EPISODE 40

STRUGGLE FOR LIFTING LOCKDOWNS

Lockdowns were easy to impose. During March and April 2020, faced with the deadly Covid-19 pandemic, almost the entire world went under lockdowns of varied durations and intensities. Some countries, especially in Europe and Americas moved with somewhat uncertainty or hesitancy—and, therefore, suffered larger loss of human life than several East-Asian countries that faced the great pandemic a lot more successful and lighter loss of human life.

Four to eight weeks of lockdowns in different countries paralyzed their economies, on one hand, and caused serious tensions and stress amongst people, young and old, who had to keep themselves to the limited space of their homes, on the other. It had raised stress in several cases and innumerable people needed help for dealing with mental imbalances resulting from the same. Domestic violence too was reported to have risen in several societies. *People couldn't be kept locked up for longer period as it raised possibilities of social conflict and public unrest.*

Consequently, governments started deliberating on lifting of lockdowns and the intricacies involved right from middle of April 2020. China was the first to lift the lockdown in Wuhan after keeping a large population locked up for over 70 days—and by the 4th week of the month almost normal movement of people, transports and functioning of businesses was restored. Taiwan, South Korea, and Vietnam had lifted restrictions on movement of people much earlier and with relative ease.

At end of April 2020, New Zealand, a small country of just five million people declared that the country was now free of the deadly virus. It lifted all restrictions on movements of people and business operations including beaches and sports arenas. Australia followed with the easing of lockdown and opened it beaches including the iconic Bondai water front of Sydney. People were seen running into blue waters as if they were, for long, deprived of an essential activity.

Italy and Spain went into lifting of lockdown restrictions with a lot of caution and hesitance. Spain had first lifted restrictions on construction business as social distancing maintenance was seen relatively easier in this business activity. Allowing of opening of small shops and mom and pop stores was the next move. Schools were opened with a lot more caution in a phased manner. In view of the psychological stresses developing in the locked-up society, Italy went ahead for opening up of parks and gardens on a priority basis but with some limitations of timing etc.

France had kept its pharmacies, bakeries and groceries functioning, like various other countries, all through the lockdown but it was a lot more stringent with restrictions on movement and outings by people in view of massive loss of life in its thousands of old-age care homes. Authorities here feared a second wave of the deadly virus' infection in case lockdown restrictions were eased early. Hence, it kept the lockdown clamped up right up to the 11th of May 2020.

Germany, like several other countries, had eased up opening of schools in a phased manner. China had allowed a large populace of students to take examinations that allowed the youngsters university entrance right towards end of April 2020. But social spacing requirements were strictly adhered to.

> *President Trump had exhibited maximum urgency towards lifting the lockdown restrictions on businesses and industry despite huge loss of human life in the county.*

By end of April 2020, one third of the total global Covid-19 infections were shared by USA and the loss of life there had crossed the level of 55,000 deaths. New York alone had suffered over 20,000 deaths, the largest count suffered by any city in the world at that time. President Trump's urgency for lifting of the lockdown had emerged from sharp fall in his popularity, on one hand, and exigencies of approaching November 2020, election, on the other. In line of his desperation, the stressed President had encouraged his followers in some states to agitate for immediate lifting of business restrictions. Responding to the situation, Florida state had gone ahead to open its beaches, malls, and other facilities of tourists' interests, while most others waited for the situation to improve.

UK's PM Boris Johnson who resumed his official duty after a long and serious encounter with the Covid-19, on 27th of April 2020 and immediately, through a press briefing, stressed that the lockdown was not to be lifted in any dangerous hurry. He feared that a second wave of the deadly virus in event of any hurry towards lifting of restrictions could push the situation out of control. Loss of human life in UK had risen to over 25,000 (including those in old-age care homes) and over a hundred of its doctors and nurses, the frontline warriors, had lost their lives while caring for others. Hence, there was a sense of scare in the country where shortage of PPEs and other life-saving necessities had created a grim scenario.

> *The struggle for lifting up of restrictions continued all through the pandemic period of 2020 and 2021—and the countries that hurried up, or where needed disciple in regard to face masking, social distancing and personal sanitation was lax, suffered resurgences of varied intensities.*

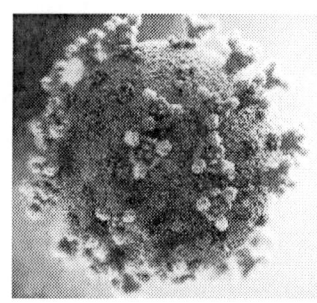

EPISODE 41

SUPPRESSION OF INFECTION AND MORTALITY DATA

The great Covid-19 pandemic scared most governments into suppression and/or hiding of infection and mortality related data. They feared that high figures in this regard would damage their standing and endanger (a) their political stability and (b) chances of re-election. It wasn't that only the elected ones harboured such fears, the autocratic ones too were no exception. Perception (rather than reality) and reputation was important for all of them.

> *The process of suppression of infection and mortality data started right from Wuhan, the birthplace of the deadly virus in China. Months later, and after a lot of international criticism, the Chinese government revised these figures which initially were kept unacceptably low.*

Coming to Southern Europe, where the deadly virus had the most vicious run in the months of March and April 2020; the affected countries were no exception to suppression of infection and deaths data. Italy, Spain, and France, the three major initial victims of Corona too were foxed into exhibiting this tendency. Possibly, it wasn't a deliberate attempt on their part because figures of infection and mortality were revised there as the pandemic progressed.

Except, possibly, Bhutan, Taiwan and New Zealand there was no other country in the world that didn't exhibited this tendency. Mismanagement of age-care homes, amongst others, had complicated and confused the infection and mortality data related situation in several western countries.

Across the channel, UK too exhibited the same tendency. But in none of the four European cases, there was any visibility of deliberate attempt to hide and/or suppress the subject data.

> *But situation was a lot different in Russia where right from the beginning, the Covid-19 related situation didn't seem transparent. When the pandemic struck, President Putin was already stressed a great deal on account of depressed crude oil prices that had crippled the Russian economy. And the country's readiness to face the situation in relation to hospital beds and ICUs, on one hand and provision of PPEs and ventilators etc, on the other, was in no way at a satisfactory level.*

At one stage Russia had responded to Italian cry for help and had sent there a team of medical personnel and some protective equipment in order to help out the heavily Covid-19 stressed country. And at that time, the autocratic dispensation didn't estimate that a crippling blast of the pandemic will blow into Moscow and other towns of the country. Soon, the autocratic regime's neck was in a constrictive grip of the dreaded Covid-19. Hospitals in Moscow had long lines of ambulances eager to off-load their cargo of Covid-19 patients. Soon, the situation suggested that things weren't transparent; there were more infections and deaths than what was being reported. And by end of May 2020, Russia pushed itself into the second highest position in the world in terms of reported infections even though there wasn't adequate testing and tracing operation in this highly stressed country.

SUPPRESSION OF INFECTION AND MORTALITY DATA

Attention on testing and tracing was most likely kept subdued so that the figure of people infected by the dreaded virus stayed low. But soon the community spread of the disease lifted curtains in a manner that things couldn't be kept under wrap any more. The communist regime was seen being helpless in its fight against the invisible enemy.

In UK too, the British government struggled for months to reach its targeted level of 1,00,000 tests every day. Finally, the target was reached but, in the meantime, by end of April 2020, it had achieved the distinction of having the highest number of Corona related deaths in the world after that of the USA. Later, Russia and Brazil had shifted UK down from this position. Prime Minister, Boris Johnson himself had suffered at hands of the great Covid-19 and was put out of functioning for over four weeks.

> *Across the Atlantic, USA too had run into a great testing and tracing controversy despite tall claims made by the Trump administration that everyone who wanted a testing will get one.*

New York, the greatest business hub of the superpower, was being mercilessly decimated by the dreaded pandemic. The great US testing and tracing deficiency controversy died down only when another great controversy related to the death of an African American named George Floyd at hands of white policemen had filled most roads and squares in USA by anti-racism related protesters. That the *'Black Lives Matter'* agitation in USA had become its largest in modern history—and it had subdued the Corona related controversies in the great country.

> *India, the largest democracy of the world that in months of March and April 2020, had consistently glorified itself for its great lockout success, too fell into a great testing and tracing related controversy.*

Consistent and deliberate efforts were made there to keep the testing efforts low. In Mumbai, Ahmedabad, and Delhi, all the three state governments, governing these business and trade hubs of the country were seen consistently suppressing the need for testing. A large number of people in front of Delhi's hospitals were seen demanding that they be tested to confirm whether they suffered with the dangerous Covid-19, but hospitals and labs intentionally refused to do the needful. Obviously, there were instructions not to test the suspected people so that the number of confirmed cases didn't rise to a level that was uncomfortable to the governing dispensations. Initially, UP, Bihar and numerous other states had totally ignored the need for testing of Corona suspected people. Their logic was simple, and the Central Government in Delhi too closed its otherwise discriminating eyes. Despite the mischief, Covid-19 infections were fast rising in India pushing it to a high level in the world just behind USA, Brazil, and Russia by the end of the 2nd week of June 2020.

In South American and African countries there was hardly any country that didn't make covert and/or overt effort to suppress testing and tracing. Situation in Brazil and Peru grew truly distressing despite governments' efforts there to hide the rampage of the dreaded pandemic. *In brief, the testing and tracing avoidance efforts of governments had become a rule rather than an exception.* And as time progressed, the situation wasn't seen improving in relation to this deliberate mischief on part of governing dispensations in major parts of the world.

* * *

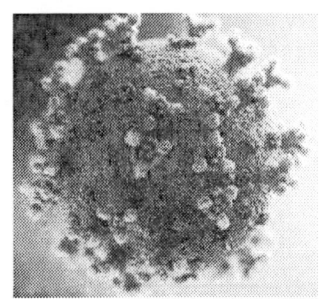

EPISODE 42

SURGE OF CORRUPTION IN COVID TIMES

Except some countries in Europe, most governments resorted to enhancing controls on various aspects of citizens' life. More controls meant less transparency and resultant greater corruption in various government activities.

There were innumerable instances of substandard PPEs procured which gave way when frontline staff attempted to put them on. In one instance in Gujarat (India) even fake ventilators were supplied by a firm that had contacts at the highest level in the state.

Indian Railways had announced that the migrant workers who were transported to their home states in most inefficient, rather horrific way, were charged for tickets by it, as well as its agents which amounted to nothing other than blatant corruption. Announcements were made by the governments that migrants' travel was free as the same was born by the state. After promising to supply food and water to the migrant workers in the trains, no such supplies were made as expected at least twice a day. Whatsoever supplies materialised—they were stale and substandard. Obviously, contractors made money at cost of the poor labours some of whom, including women and children, died for want of food and water.

> *Most governments made emergency purchases of PPE kits, testing kits, masks, drugs, ventilators, and other ICU needs in the Covid times and, as per assessment of the author, none of these was free of cuts pocketed by those responsible for the purchase process.*

It was true for India and most other developing and under-developed countries in the third world. And hence, the inbuilt corruption in the system of governance was responsible, at least in part, for higher casualties at hands of the pandemic and the widely visible disregard and disrespect to even the dead.

> *Supplies of free/subsidized rations in India to poor ration card holders, in the Covid times, were hugely adulterated and fungus infested that, in many cases, even animals refused to eat the same when offered as feed.*

State governments that supposedly made arrangements for quarantine etc for arriving streams of labourers failed miserably in making such arrangements, including supply of food and water; corruption was visible in all aspects of handling of movements of the migrating workers. People suffered and died in times of Covid-19 like flies and government officials and their agents indulged in corruption in most inhuman manner.

> *And the author is sure that India wasn't the only case in the world for such corruptions on part of incompetent authorities. Numerous inefficient governances in Asia, Africa and South American countries behaved in similar manner.*

Thus, Covid-19 had generated huge opportunities for blatant corruption.

* * *

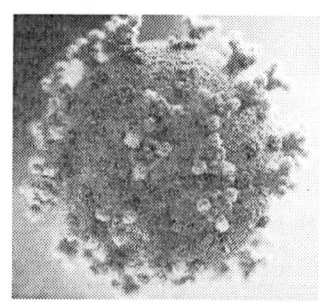

EPISODE 43

CONFLICT BETWEEN SAVING LIVES AND PROTECTING LIVELIHOOD

> *When Covid-19 struck the mankind in the first quarter of 2020, the first response of the deeply stressed multitude of countries was to save lives i.e., to isolate and quarantine the infected, treat those who were infected and lockout the rest—and thus attempting to limit spread of the deadly virus.*

Priority of governments changed as time passed. This invisible enemy of the humanity grew in an exponential manner and thus had potential to infect most of the world population before either the so-developed herd immunity discouraged further spread of the disease or application of vaccines intervened in some effective manner.

Almost every government in the world, as herd behaviour, opted for imposing lockouts—closing most businesses and human interactions, including industries, and restricting movement of goods and services. But the virus possibly was more intelligent than human-beings; it multiplied amongst the locked-up population because the much touted social or physical distancing wasn't always possible. Care homes, ill-equipped hospitals, and cramped-up residences which housed several persons per room helped the pathogen to breed unabatedly. *Millions died, mortuaries were filled, and burial grounds fell short of space.* Mass graves became the resting place of the unfortunates who came in the path of the dreaded virus. In most cases burial and/or funeral rituals were given a go by. People not only died lonely death and were buried while no one was around to shed a tear. It was a horrifying situation that the mankind had no memory of having witnessed such a situation in the past.

In the avalanche of Corona, jobs were lost like leaves drop in fall season—and soon affected families ran short of money for essentials, even for putting food on the table. By end of May 2020, the situation had become truly horrible.

> *Questions were raised whether the Corona was a bigger enemy or the lockdowns that were supposed to arrest its deadly march. Economy and livelihoods were gasping for air and new normal were crowding the space for adoption by the hugely tormented mankind for its survival.*

The second concern that had overshadowed the first seemed that people now argued whether saving livelihoods was more important in the situation since hungry, isolated, and depressed people were an easier prey for the deadly virus to grab and strangulate. President Trump of USA and Jair Bolsonaro of Brazil were the most active advocates of this approach.

Two to three months' long lockdowns clamped in most of the countries of the world had starved their economies for vital revenues and taxes, on one hand and enhanced expenditures incurred in fighting the dreaded disease emptied exchequers, on the other. Most countries pushed their central banks for greater liquidity and many others approached the IMF for loans. Some resorted to monetizing valued assets, reducing social welfare spending and shedding other avoidable expenses.

In case of all major and medium economies of the world GDPs fell without exception; some contracted by 10-25 percent and even more. In brief, there was economic chaos all around and an environment of depression just waited on margins to overtake. Predictions about economic situations for the next 2-3 years offered no great hopes of relief.

The lockouts of varied durations (mostly lasting 5-10 weeks) resorted to by most of the countries in the pandemic ravaged world didn't turn out to be a Brahmastra against the cunning virus; they only slowed down the pathogen and lengthened its span of devastation. The lockdowns caused to stop functioning of most businesses and industry except for (a) medical infrastructure that fought the pandemic (though not with great successes), and (b) bureaucracies assisted by security forces who implemented the lockdowns. As a result, 85-90 percent of the working populations were rendered unemployed during the period. Some worked from home, yet productivity died down, GDPs nose-dived, and state exchequers started drying up. Businesses expressed inability to pay wages to so idled work force.

> *In India the dreaded second wave of the pandemic in April/May 2021 pushed a quarter of its population (additional to the existing one huge number in this category) below the poverty line. Ninety seven percent pf the population lost incomes in varying amounts. But the government thought of no relief except providing 4-5 kg of grains to over 800 million people for some months.*

Some governments in the west had, however, willingly come forward to pay wages to the so idled employees, most through compensation to their employers and some directly through cash transfers. But the effort was just a drop in the ocean, on one hand and crippled the struggling state finances, on the other.

> *In India, an over 400 million strong work force (including those in the informal sector) was turned unemployed in a crude stroke of thoughtless governance.*

Incomes of the so unemployed work force weren't protected. Soon migrant workers holed up in small windowless dwellings could not pay rent and were evicted by landlords. And the 21 days (initially supposed duration) lockdown that started on 24th March 2020 with just 4 hours' notice was extended three times. As a consequence, the homeless and aimless work force that was holed up in over a hundred industrial and business hubs scattered all over the country started moving out to go to their villages. They found themselves in a precarious situation as road and rail transport in the country was in lockdown. Huge masses of migrant workers assembled on bus stations and finding that the governments (state as well as the one at the centre) didn't bother for them, started walking on foot on national and state highways. Police harassed them and many of them died walking, hungry and thirsty. The Chaos continued for almost three summer months when temperatures soared to high forties.

> *Continents away in USA, over 40 million had registered for unemployment benefits and salary restorations. In Europe too almost all countries, in one or the other way, took care of income of people who were rendered jobless by the great pandemic and human reaction to it in form of lockdowns.*

Lengthening lines of hungry in front of soup kitchen, food banks and lungers (the Indian mode of food charities) illustrated the stressed situation caused by the pandemic and its aftermath. And the situation didn't improve as the Covid year 2020 drew to closure.

Covid-19 and the lockdowns which were erroneously thought as cure for the pandemic, caused irreparable damage to economies, national as well as international. When hugely stressed governments wanted to lift lockdowns and open up economies, many businesses struggled to stand-up. While some commenced work with reduced work force and scaled down capacities, several of them filed for protection under respective states' bankruptcy laws.

The businesses and industries related to travel, tourism and hospitality including, aviation (airlines as well as aircraft manufactures), hotel and restaurant chains suffered the most. Many of these and related businesses asked for bailouts; some survived on LORR owed oxygen and a lot many collapsed to the ground never to rise again.

> *In the conflict between saving lives and livelihoods governments first attempted to save lives but failed or only partly succeeded—and then, starved for revenues, scaled down the effort in favour of saving livelihoods in an unorganised and confused manner. In final analysis most governments failed in resolving both or any one of the conflicting objectivities.*

* * *

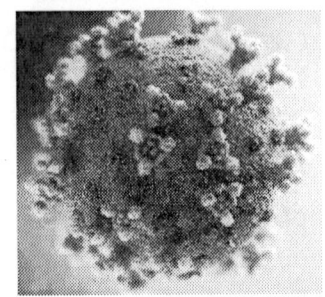

EPISODE 44

TRUTH BECAME THE GREATEST CASUALTY OF COVID-19 PANDEMIC

Covid-19 killed millions of people in the world right in the first year of its rampage—and the actual number of its killings was said to be much higher than that reported by various governments and collated by the WHO etc. Some governments weren't worried that so many people died—they were worried about the factual situation going viral and the same damaging credibility of those involved in governance and/or mis-governance.

> *USA suffered maximum casualties—by middle of the first quarter of the 2021; it had lost over 5,00,000 people that exceeded its losses in the Vietnam combined with the 1st and the 2nd WWs.*

Right in the beginning when the dreaded pandemic raised its head in Wuhan, the Chinese authorities suppressed information (a) about its origin, and (b) also about its severity or killing potential. WHO, by design or otherwise, became a part of the Chinese misinformation drive in regard to the deadly pandemic.

> *But the greatest casualty of information related truth at hands of the killer virus occurred in India, Russia Brazil where political dispensations were more scared of the adverse publicity that the great pathogen could bring if correct numbers of dead were disclosed.*

Some other countries such as Pakistan, Iran, and Turkey too exhibited similar tendencies at relatively lower scale. None of these countries displaying love for hiding data in regard to people infected by the virus and those who became victims, was short of people and for these governments a few thousand deaths, this or that way, were indeed immaterial—but what they feared most was the information going viral.

India with over 1,300 million people exhibited its intensions regarding hiding data related to people infected and those who became victim of the pandemic in several ways. Firstly, the publicity loving Government of India while imposing an unplanned lockout on 24th March 2020 had claimed that it would overwhelm the virus just in 18 days like it had defeated evil forces at Kurukshetra some 5,000 years ago. It extended the lockdown three times and when Indian economy tanked, it hurried up with lifting of restrictions in an unplanned and messy manner.

Secondly, it didn't seriously follow WHO advice about testing; its testing facilities were inadequate and of uncertain quality. Millions of testing kits that were imported haphazardly through corrupt middlemen from China had to be returned. And preparations towards upgrading facilities in hospitals in regard to Covid beds i.e., with oxygen, ventilators and PPEs etc were lousy. Its prime emphasis was more on publicity than on performance.

> *It thought that good and sustained publicity could whitewash everything.*

It took a lot of time in allowing private labs to go for creating testing facilities and then (possibly deliberately) kept testing fee payable by individuals so high that only few could afford. By early May 2020, growing infection in Mumbai, Chennai, Ahmedabad and Delhi unnerved the government into issuing several misleading and contradictory guidelines to state governments in regards to testing, tracing and quarantining etc. And the same were altered frequently.

Everyone who wanted a test couldn't get one since the procedure was bureaucratic and hence discouraged people to come forward. The unstated logic perhaps was that less testing will bring lower numbers of infections to light and deaths occurring due to the pandemic could always be assigned to co-morbidities or pre-existing diseases.

*In numerous cases, the cause of death in certificates of Covid patients was listed as **'respiratory failure'**.* Doctors and other frontline workers informally confirmed that the number of people who fell to the dreaded pandemic was much higher than officially reported.

In April 2020, health ministry of the Central Government started with daily press conference to give out details of those found infected by the virus and also those who were killed by it in previous 24 hours. There was tendency to highlight figures related to opposition ruled states and minimised for those governed by its own party and its allies.

When situation related to growing infections and deaths became serious by May 2020, conducting such conferences became first infrequent and then stopped totally. It wasn't without anti-people intentions.

> *Several misinformation and fake news were promoted by the pro-government TV channels and print media stating that the Corona will meet its waterloo in India (a) due to its summer heat, (b) helped by the younger population, and (c) practice of BCG vaccination etc.*

GOI's Ayush ministry too promoted several untruths about efficacy of herbal concoctions. On 23rd June 2020, a government friendly yoga guru launched an ayurvedic formulation named **'Coronil'** for treatment of Covid-19 without any confirmatory tests and/or approvals from appropriate authorities. No one seemed to question the launch of a doubtful formulation, except some in the medical fraternity.

And pro-government army of astrologers, pundits and tantric's too went berserk promoting untruths and, thus, misleading people through government friendly TV channels and social media.

While the pandemic assumed tsunami like proportions in June/July 2020, government spokesmen consistently denied that a community transmission of the virus had occurred in India. People were now scared and didn't know whom to trust. How many people were killed by the deadly pandemic seemed much higher than those reported by the government. Situation in hospital wards and at funeral centres weren't considered and collated truthfully.

> *Russian data in regard to infections and deaths reported were never trustable. The autocratic regime had deep interest in not allowing rest of the world know the true situation.*

What was the truth about persistent shortage of PPE kits and beds in hospitals can never be known. And did some frontline workers in hospitals who expressed dissatisfaction with the situation jumped out of windows willingly or were they pushed out to silence them, shall never be known.

Brazil was another typical country where truth about the degree of infection and the number of people dying at hands of the deadly virus had become a casualty. Looking at the graveyards and freshly dug graves there and also the conditions in hospital wards went to suggest that the reported figures of Covid-19 infections and deaths had no relation to what had actually happened.

In case of USA, President Trump's disconnection with the truth in regard to the Covid-19 had become crystal clear by end of May 2020, when he aggressively encouraged and advocated opening-up of the deeply distressed businesses and industry. His recourse to untruths was understandable considering (a) his basic nature of discordant communication, and (b) compulsions related to his re-election plans in November 2020. Several experts' deposition before

Congress, in relation to Covid-19 and related aspects, had established beyond doubts that truth was the greatest casualty of the deadly pandemic in the oldest democracy of the world.

> *These are just the major example where truth had become the major casualty at hands of Covid-19—but the list of countries where truth suffered a great deal was, in fact, fairly large.*

And this trend of untruth propagation by various governments continued unabated all through the deadly run of the Covid-19 during 2020 and 2021 and even afterwards.

* * *

EPISODE 45

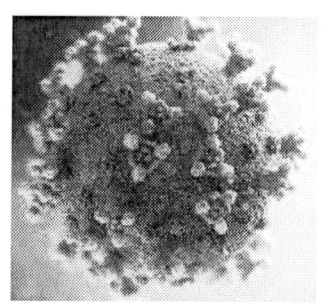

UNCERTAINTIES THROWN UP BY THE CORONAVIRUS

There were several uncertainties and non-understandings about this dreaded disease. As time passed and world's medical fraternity gained experience in dealing with the virus, the scenario of complications expanded progressively. Some of the main ones included:

1. Firstly, the origin of Coronavirus was clouded with uncertainties. Whether it was of natural origin or a product of human mischief remained wholly uncertain—and this riddle may never be solved. Americans called it as a *"Chinese Virus"* implying that it was a Chinese mischief thrown at the humanity. A WHO team of experts landed in Wuhan towards end of January 2021 but nothing much came out of it because of Chinese reluctance to cooperate.

2. It was also alleged that the Coronavirus might have been an attempt to create and test a biological tool or weapon for the purpose of attaining an unassailable superiority in event of conflict. This unique weapon would have allowed attacking an adversary, or a group of them, without entering their territory from ground and/or air.

3. Chinese wild animals' market near Wuhan and sale of bats there for human consumption was suspected to be the source from where this deadly virus escaped. But no confirmation has been possible.
4. It has been difficult to differentiate between the Coronavirus caused symptoms and those of the normal flu infections. Its nature of initial un-symptomatic presence in patients caused considerable uncertainties as well as massive anxiety.
5. What works and what doesn't towards minimising intensity of Covid-19 infections have never been clear. Whether Hydroxy Chloroquine (HCQ) gave some relief against the deadly disease remained an area of total uncertainties.
6. Whether Covid-19 spreads only through droplets that come out while sneezing and/or coughing by patients or it can jump through air from an infected person to a non-infected one, couldn't be determined with certainties during initial months of its spread despite all the technology available to human-beings.
7. Whether one could safely go out for a walk, or resort to outdoor cycling, for needed exercise remained uncertain for a long time.
8. For how long can the Covid-19 infection survive on plastic, steel, wood, cloth and all other type of surfaces which humans normally encounter in day-to-day activities remained unclear. Even newspapers were looked upon as suspect and sales of the same nose-dived during the pandemic period.
9. Whether after an individual was declared negative after a test, was he/she wholly free of remains of Civid-19 continued in doubt. And why re-emergence of the disease took place in some individuals and not in others continued as a riddle.
10. Whether the hot or cold weather conditions mattered for multiplication and spread of the virus had caused confusion for a long time.

11. The need and/or utility of wearing a face mask for checking spread of this virus too remained disputed. Several leaders contributed to this confusion despite experts' clear opinion in its favour.

12. What kind of negative after-effects this pandemic was likely to leave behind on human society and/or its economic activities remained uncertain—more like the situation that is often left after an earthquake.

13. Long and short-term after-effects of the pathogen on various parts of human body (after initial recovery of patients) continued to bother the medical experts and some hospitals went ahead to open post-Covid-19 advice and care centres as recovered persons continued to voice lingering complaints.

14. Covid-19 threw education, at all levels from primary to university, out of gear. Annual examinations were postponed and entrance tests to medical and engineering colleges ran into trouble. The whole student community suffered dreadful stress on this account.

15. Maximum uncertainties were encountered in the field of economy were reopening up complications, loss of jobs and incomes had affected a large section of population almost in all countries. Several governments ran short of revenues and struggled even for continuing their basic governance activities.

16. Mutations of the virus, British as well as non-British ones caused massive anxiety and uncertainties. How far will vaccines succeed against it in time to come?

As the Covid year 2020 gave way to 2021, new uncertainties about the dreaded virus continued to emerge. In author's opinion, there shall never be total clarity in regard to this bio-agent and the chaos that it created.

* * *

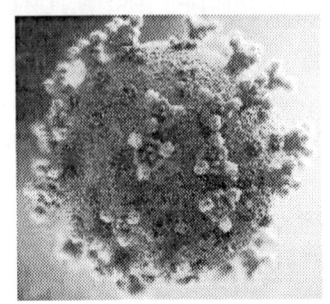

EPISODE 46

CORONA: A FAST UNFOLDING SCENARIO

Middle of April 2020, Dr Anthony Fauci of CDC had opined that the US President delayed initiating measures to fight the Corona and a lot many lives could have been saved if preventive measures were taken in time. President Trump exhibited displeasure at the unpleasant observation but refrained from firing the famous scientist. Further, some other experts had opined that deaths from the Corona Virus infections were substantially under-reported in several countries, including USA. Fear of political repercussions had weighed heavily on the so erring governments. Care-homes' deaths from Europe as well as USA were being underreported because old resident could neither practice physical distancing nor were, they free from pre-existing conditions. They fell quick prey to the virus and in several cases these deaths were passed as normal event.

> Dr Gopinath of IMF had opined that the world GDP in 2020 shall shrink to minus three percent and was unlikely to recover during the year. By the year end, the economic damage caused by the Corona turned out much more serious. And improvements in 2021 looked uncertain.

Medical staff in almost all countries of the world was seen

struggling with the inadequacy of PPEs and related tools, including drugs to deal with the situation thrown up by the pandemic.

Several doctors, other health care workers and experts reported off camera that India wasn't testing enough and also under-reported Corona infections as well as deaths that it caused. A similar situation prevailed in several countries, especially in the developing world. Not admitting the sick and infected to hospitals too was reported often and people were seen dying waiting in ambulances.

> *President Trump (mid-April 2020) had suspended financial assistance to the WHO for (a) not doing its job well enough, and (b) extending opinion against suspension of air travel to and from China in the 1st quarter of 2020—thus having helped in spreading infection world over.*

South Korea went through an election effectively employing physical distancing, on one hand and implementing usage of masks and gloves etc, on the other. Experts opined that East Asian countries like South Korea, Taiwan, Vietnam, Singapore and Japan did a better job of testing and containment than the developed countries in the West.

As the Covid year 2020 gave way to 2021, the scenario caused by the dreaded virus grew darker despite rush of several vaccines with a promise of relief to the hugely stressed mankind.

Towards middle of 2021 several Covid associated diseases, most prominent of which was black fungus, and the fear of third wave in India had complicated the scenario.

* * *

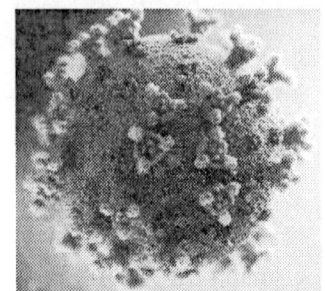

EPISODE 47

USA LANDED IN DEADLY GRIP OF CORONA

USA, in the initial period of Coronavirus outbreak in China and then its fast spread to other East-Asian countries like South Korea, Japan, Taiwan, Malaysia and Singapore, didn't take the Corona disease seriously. It called Corona as the *'Chinese Virus'* and on 11th March 2020, when WHO declared it as a Pandemic, President Trump took it light-heartedly and, as a consequence, the Superpower didn't start planning its defences seriously. By the time total infections in the world were just above a 1,00,000 even though deaths in Italy, Spain and Iran were crippling the total medical infrastructure of these nations, USA continued to ignore the threat.

> *Since the trans-Atlantic air travel was not restricted, the deadly virus took an easy ride to all over North as well as South American continents. The critical load of the pathogen reaching USA was high because a major part of the air traffic to the new world was destined to US cities or passed through the same.*

It was reported that a senior White House functionary (the trade advisor to the President) had warned the US administration through a memo which stated that USA could lose millions of lives to the deadly Covid-19 and that its economy might suffer trillions of US$

damages. The warning was sadly ignored and even a repeat submission wasn't paid attention. The President was busy planning his India visit and negotiate a large trade deal. The India visit took place on 24 and 25 February 2020, though the anticipated trade agreement didn't come through. A deal worth US$ 2.6 billion for supplying some helicopters to India did come through—and the President had a memorable photo opportunity with Taj in the background at Agra. Another take-away of the visit was *"Namaste"*, the Indian system of greeting visitors. Later, it came handy to the President in promoting social distancing when the Covid-19 had taken a devastating grip on several cities of USA.

By 11th April or just before the Easter Sunday, USA had become the world's largest casualty; its Corona deaths count in New York itself had run into several thousands. Total cases of infections in US had risen to half a million. The world had suffered over a 1,00,000 deaths, Italy, Spain, and USA leading the tally.

> *On a single day USA had registered over 2100 deaths–half of which came from New-York alone. Several of the US cities were in deadly grip of the so-called Chinese virus. US medical infrastructure was now cracking under the load of Corona infections. Hospitals and other medical facilities ran short of PPEs and ventilators. Though the President claimed that there wasn't any need for putting masks, but the country ran short of this simple device too and people resorted to home-made devices.*

Orders for import of PPEs and ventilators were put on numerous local, as well as foreign firms but supplies took time to arrive and to get distributed to different states. Doctors and nurses were seen improvising for the protective devices and numerous of these frontline workers caught infection. Several of them died too in their un-equal fight against the deadly Corona.

There were more African Americans and Hispanics amongst the sick and dead; the Corona preferred to have them as victims in proportion of 3 : 1 as the jobs they normally did were riskier and more devoid of safety.

> *The situation grew so serious in the iconic city of New-York that huge field hospitals had to be erected in parks at a breakneck speed and staff to man the same had to be gathered by calling in the retired doctors and nurses.*

Corona was merciless; it seemed as if the pandemic was taking a revenge on the world's Superpower for being ignored by its President in the initial months of the new year, or he calling it as a *"Chinese Virus".*

The deadly Corona hadn't spared even an iconic US aircraft career stationed at Guam. Responding to the challenge, US navy had to station a medical services ship near the threatened city of New York, in river Hudson. The Superpower also seemed to have run out of medicines at one stage to treat its sick—and the beleaguered President was seen threatening India if it didn't allow export of the HCQ and other essential drugs needed by US. And India promptly gave in to the threat.

> *The Superpower found it difficult to handle its dead. Dead bodies were stored in refrigerated vans as morgues were full to their neck. It resorted to mass burial of the dead at the 'heart island' in six feet deep mass graves.*

In May and June 2020, the Corona had spread to all the 50 US states and the country had achieved the distinction of being the only country in the world that had suffered over 2.5 million infections and 1,25,000 deaths. The Superpower was on the mat and its irrational President's discordant ways and differences with top US experts had contributed a great deal to the hopeless situation. President Trump's attempts to open up the US economy in May and June had brought in a punishing resurgence of the deadly virus by end of June 2020.

The great nation was again on the mat while the dreaded virus stood its ground mocking at it vigorously. And, in the process, President Trump was put firmly on path to losing the November 2020 re-election.

The dreaded Corona kept resurging in various states and the ones which had hurried up to open-up businesses and industries in response to President's push and cajoling were punished the most. Florida, Texas, and Arizona suffered the most. The resurgence of Corona continued all through July and August and therefore, for the first time in history, nominations as presidential candidates for the upcoming elections by both the contending parties were done without crowds and usual applauses. Corona was seen killing the election game.

'Black Lives Matter' demonstrations that continued for over two months in July and August, came handy for the Corona virus to spread its wings far and wide. By end of August 2020, the death toll in USA had climbed up to cross the 1,80,000 mark. As campaign for the November Presidential election heated up, Corona too continued its march unhindered.

The election happened in November and Trump lost the fight, but Corona wasn't tired in any way and it continued to devastate various population centres of the Superpower totally unhindered. The Christmas and New Year festivities remained substantially subdued. Only an aggressive vaccination campaign that commenced in Mid-December brought some hopes for relief.

By middle of the first quarter of the New Year the great Superpower had lost half a million valuable lives that exceeded the collective loss of Vietnam war and also the two world wars.

* * *

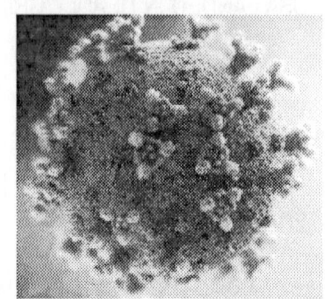

EPISODE 48

MASSIVE EFFORTS TOWARDS VACCINES' DEVELOPMENT

Since there was no effective medicine available for treatment of Covid-19, it was natural for leading scientific institutions to press for development of vaccines for encountering the vicious pandemic. Serious efforts in this regard commenced right early in the Covid year 2020. USA, UK, Russia, China, and India were seen making leading efforts in this regard. WHO and several philanthropic institutions got involved early in this vital effort and initially there was no shortage of funds needed for expediting research in this direction. The normally needed time of several years for maturing of such efforts had to be compressed into a year or even less.

Testing for safety and efficacy of emerging candidates was undertaken more or less simultaneously and, as a consequence, results started pouring in right in the third quarter of 2020. And by end of the year six vaccines namely, two from USA and one each from UK, Russia, China, and India, were ready for launch against the dreaded pandemic.

Approvals for use of these products by relevant regulatory agencies were expedited at a breakneck speed. And despite apprehensions, massive efforts to first vaccinate frontline workers in all the vaccine producing and several other countries were launched right in the first quarter of the year 2021. Rich countries made large financial provisions and attempted to corner bulk of the supplies. USA and UK took lead in this direction and WHO and some experts voiced concern against an emerging vaccine apartheid. In view of aggressive campaigns in several countries, emergence of some reluctance amongst masses to come forward and get the jab too was witnessed as misinformation through social media etc was seen confusing people. Despite limitations and apprehensions vaccination became the prime tool to fight the dreaded pandemic in 2021.

> *Corona wasn't ready to retreat in face of vaccines' combined attack; it surged, resurged, and mutated to create more vicious strains and kept on its war against mankind for a long time.*

* * *

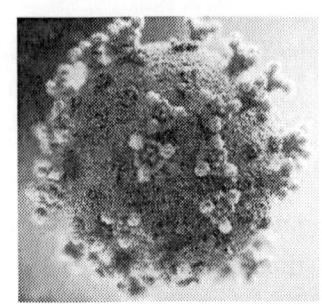

EPISODE 49

INDIA'S DISASTROUS SECOND WAVE

> *India's management of Covid pandemic was indeed a great disaster. Towards middle of April 2021 a complacent and unprepared India landed itself into the world's worst Covid-19 chaos.*

The Hindutva-stained government of Prime Minister Narendra Modi ignored experts' advice and preferred to organise elections in five states in March/April 2021. For him winning votes has been and continues to be more important than saving lives. Hence, the whole central government not only concentrated on to organising massive rallies and road shows but also declared that it had defeated the virus. Just when elections still lingered on in April people started to fall to the dreaded virus like flies do under an insecticide spray.

> *They died in their congested residences uncared for; most without medicines, oxygen and other vital medical attention. They died in their personal vehicles, taxis, 3-wheelers, ambulances and on handcarts while taking rounds of hospitals which overflowed with patients gasping for breath—and the ones already dead.*
>
> *They died in parking lots, on hospital gates and on pavements while pleading for medical attention. Dead bodies piled up in hospital corridors and in mortuaries.*

Wrapped in plastic, they formed a ghastly scenario. Crematoria and burial grounds presented scenes never witnessed in the living memory of all Indians. Fires from cremation grounds lighted dark nights in metros as well as in small towns—and flames from burning pyres could be seen from a distance. The capital city of New Delhi and towns like Gurugram, Ghaziabad, Lucknow, Varanasi, Patna, Ahmedabad and Surat, amongst others, were seen struggling to dispose-off the dead.

> *In Agra a woman, while waiting for medical attention, was seen attempting to breath in some air into mouth of her dying husband. In a Poona flat, an eighteen-month-old toddler sat crying near her dead mother, thirsty and hungry, for over two days till police rescued her on complaint of neighbours. And these weren't isolated events.*
>
> *Breakdown of centuries rich social culture was seen crumbling under the dreaded Corona's merciless avalanche.*

At some places chimneys of electric crematoria collapsed in face-of uninterrupted burning of dead bodies. Several traditional crimination grounds ran short of wood and space. Several such grounds or ghats had to add new platforms to burn dead bodies—and in New Delhi even canine burial grounds were used to deal with the flood of victims of Corona.

Amongst ghastly scenes, wait at cremation grounds was long and painful. Invariably, dead bodies lined up and grieving relatives waited up to or even beyond 24 hours with tokens and/or coupons in their hands. Well-connected and influential, however, attempted to jump the queue. Overcharging towards funeral costs became more of a rule than an exception—in some cases people paid 4-5 times that of the normal charges. And insensitive authorities looked the other way. They were busy suppressing data of dead and dying. This kind of insensitivity wasn't witnessed even during the early 20th century's **'Spanish Flu'** and *'Bengal Famine'* mismanaged by the British regime.

> *For villagers in thousands in UP and Bihar high costs of funerals and shortage of wood forced them just to toss dead bodies into the holy Ganga river.*

Additionally, several crimination ghats on the riverbanks just pushed half burnt bodies into the holy stream. Soul of Bhagiratha, the great Indian ancient king, who had toiled to bring the holy river to earth was in tears.

Some crematoria resorted to mass burning of bodies which was grossly against Hindu traditions. Situation in burial grounds wasn't any different; they ran out of space and were short of labourers to dig graves. In some cases, mass burials were resorted to. In both cases i.e., at the burning ghats as well as burial grounds normal rituals were given a go by. And often dead weren't treated with respect that was due to departing souls in the traditional Indian society.

> *In brief, it seemed that the dreaded Corona enjoyed enacting a 'naked dance of death'. It was, possibly, punishing the inadequately equipped and careless section of mankind with a sense of revenge.*

* * *

COVID-19 CATAPULTED INDIA TO STRANGE GLORY

When India was busy claiming to have grabbed the position of **'Vishva Guru'** and **'Saviour'** of the world by providing needed medicines and vaccines, the second wave of Covid-19 in middle of May 2021 pushed it to top position in the world in terms of *'highest daily reported infections and deaths'* regularly for 2-3 weeks at stretch. The following heights achieved were of significance:

1. *'Half of the daily cases of infections and a third of the daily reported deaths reported in whole world were in India'*. Every day since April 25th to 17th May more than 40 percent of reported Corona infection cases were reported from India. On some days during the period the figure touched 50 percent of the whole

world' data. WHO data showed that India reported more Covid infections than rest of the world on May 4, 5, 10, 11 and 12. Since May 4 India also reported 30 percent of global Covid deaths. And several experts had opined that actual figures were, in fact, several times higher than the reported ones.

Only other country that came close to having half of the world's cases in a day was USA. India, however, bettered US figure of 47 percent by touching a peak with 54 percent.

2. *When on peak India also achieved a positivity rate that was amongst the highest ones in the world.*

3. While vaccines saved lives in rich countries India exported available dozes to over 80 countries—and that it wasn't the right approach was debated in India for a long time. Slow vaccination had thus left India vulnerable when the disastrous second wave came to push it to a state of strange glory. *'And the world was visibly scared of Indian variants to the extent that most countries suspended travel to and fro India for the fear of the so-called variants overturning their improving Covid scenario'.*

* * *

WHAT CAUSED THE CHAOS DURING THE SECOND WAVE IN INDIA

The arrogant and insensitive government of India was caught unprepared by the clever bio-agent called Covid-19. The Hindutva-stained government was busy winning elections, arranging *'Kumbh Mela'* and promoting *'Astha'* and superstition of all types. It had grown excessively sensitive to views of any other hue than its own and also snarled at good suggestions. Its autocratic nature had blinded it from seeing factual situations on the ground—and anyone who dared to point out or complain was threatened with filing of police cases and detention under draconian laws. Differing views, political or otherwise, was brutally curbed and intellectualism of any type, other than the one related to Hindutva, was viewed as a threat to its existence.

In middle of May 2021, when Aam Admi Party (AAP) in New Delhi put an innocuous poster that questioned government's vaccine policy, FIRs were filed against labourers who were employed to stick the said bills. It exhibited the Indian government's total lack of tolerance even to simple forms of criticism which is essential for survival of democracy.

Indian government didn't take advantage of the long window that was allowed by the Corona virus between the first and second wave to enhance investments towards mending the country's crumbling healthcare infrastructure. It deliberately curbed operations of opposition ruled states by denying funds due to them. Funds were wasted on avoidable projects such as a *'new central vista'* in New Delhi as a mark of prestige—and also on purchasing hugely costly planes for travel of its top leaders. It also wasted fund on security of its B-grade leaders and hangers-on. It looked to sensitive observers that lives of common man didn't matter while dividing people on religious grounds, raising new temples, and erecting huge statues to fool people and garner votes was its top priority. Blatant untruth and false propaganda were resorted to for covering up its misdeeds of omission and commission.

* * *

THE GREAT INDIAN OXYGEN EMERGENCY

In April and May 2021, a massive spurt of Covid for a period of 4 to 5 weeks threw hospitals in Delhi, Gurugram, Lucknow, Patna, Jaipur, Mumbai, Ahmedabad, Surat, Bengaluru, Chennai and several other metros and towns into an unprecedented chaos of deaths and desperation. No Covid beds with oxygen and ventilators were available and only a few lucky patients who had high level of contacts could get into ICUs. It caused massive oxygen demand by hospitals and also by individuals who were isolating in their homes. Several suffering hospitals and a few state governments approached Supreme Court of India and High courts for more reliable supply. The central government was responsible for allocating oxygen to various states and on having no clear answers or plans to meet the surging demand the frustrated judiciary castigated government regularly for weeks during relevant hearings.

While persisting shortage of oxygen killed innumerable patients in hospitals and in-home isolation, India's health minister Dr. Harsh Vardhan was seen repeatedly claiming on TV channels that there was no shortage of oxygen in the country. It was the **'greatest lie of the new century'** as at almost the same time the Modi government had pleaded with foreign governments to rush oxygen, essential medicines and breathing equipment to India. Similarly, the Chief Minister of UP, India's most populous state, persistently claimed that there wasn't shortage of any type, hospital beds and/or oxygen. Even while people died like flies outside hospitals and in parking grounds, several high-level government functionaries didn't desist from uttering and spreading blatant untruth. And those who complained on social media were threatened with filing of FIRs and arrest. These weren't isolated cases since a large number of BJP led government functionaries made insensitive and shameless claims and comments. They seemed confused and didn't know how to face truth on the ground. For them a few hundred thousand or even million deaths didn't make a difference.

Bureaucracy, the essential wheels of governance in New Delhi, had long stopped making independent public-interest related decisions. Constitutional bodies like judiciary, election commission, information commission of India, RBI, CBI, CAG etc., which were earlier viewed independent and had kept the Indian democracy on its rails, were pushed into submission and now towed the Hindutva-stained government's lines. Planning Commission of India was disbanded, and no system of governance was left operative truthfully—and hence no one had seen the dreaded Corona avalanche (the second wave) coming the country's way.

The medical emergency so caused by the second wave of Corona in the April and May 2021 was indeed unprecedented. Thousands of patients died in several well-known hospitals. One hospital in Agra deliberately stopped oxygen supply to patients to determine who needed it most—and two dozen of them died within minutes. One expert in Maharashtra opined that 25 percent of deaths in the deadly 2nd wave had occurred on account of oxygen supply failures. No other country, small or big, developed or otherwise, had faced such a painful situation. The dreaded virus had taken advantage of lack of planning on part of the government of India that was lulled into complacency when the pandemic had receded in 4th quarter of the Covid year 2020. It had gone into election mode creating numerous super-spreading events, on one hand and singing its own praise as how it had performed better than several developed countries in face of the pandemic, on the other. Huge amount of funds were spent on publicity in order to misguide the public about its non-existent successes and achievements. Manipulating public perceptions with a view to garner votes and enabling the Hindutva-stained BJP to win in West Bengal, Assam, Tamil Nadu, Kerala, and Puducherry elections. Employing huge funds at its disposal and also the misuse of ED, CBI and several other central agencies, it engineered defections from opposition parties, especially in West Bengal. Its priorities were grossly misplaced.

It also ran into an overdrive to export vaccines, Covid relevant drugs and medical oxygen to several countries and claimed through Indian media (controlled by BJP money bags) that it had saved the world from the pandemic. It forgot the fact that Covid was still around and could attack viciously at time of its choice. In the process, it ignored experts' opinion and decided not to plan defences against the dreaded pandemic. When a regrouped, well-rested and hugely mutated Corona re-attacked in the 2nd fortnight of April 2021, the arrogant and non-performing government was caught pants down. Confused and disoriented by the vicious second wave, it resorted to blaming opposition ruled states of negligence and lack of action. But that wasn't enough of a defence and soon deficiencies on its part were well in the open for everyone to see. An enraged Corona struck hard and wide taking almost whole the country in its grip, creating the world record in terms of daily reported cases of infections (over 4 lakh new infections every day for over two weeks without a break and also around 4,000 or more daily reported deaths. This time the great virus also decided to walk into rural India where no functional medical infrastructure of any type existed. Unreported loss of life including that in rural areas was put around 4-5 (and some experts had put the same at 7, 10, 15, 20 and 25 times higher) times of the reported figures. Medical infrastructure collapsed, running short of beds, ICUs, oxygen, and drugs almost all over the country.

> *Doctors and nurses grew desperate and some of them were seen in tears on account of their inability to save valuable lives.*

Though not admitting the fact, the government of India panicked and made desperate appeal for assistance from foreign countries to rush essential drugs, ventilators, oxygen, and equipment to generate and transport the lifesaving input. The self-proclaimed **'Vishva Guru'** and supplier of vaccines to several dozen countries unprecedentedly turned into an international bagger.

* * *

PANDEMIC EXPOSED INDIA'S COVID-19 FAULT-LINES

Astha (blinding religious faith and practices), elections and numerous festivals are India's Covid related fault-lines. It is unfortunate that the Indian government failed to understand and appreciate the danger posed by the deadly fault-lines which, in time of the second Covid wave, led to massive loss of human lives and incalculable adverse impacts on the society.

India had unwisely claimed that it managed Covid-19 outbreak of 2020 better than several developed countries.

The autocratic governance had ignored to see the potential danger when Covid had slowed down in the 4th quarter of 2020 and the first one of the New Year. It was busy claiming credit that, in fact, didn't belong to it. The fault-lines on the Indian scenario exploded when a well-rested and regrouped Covid viciously attacked and caused the 2nd wave during the 2nd quarter of 2021. Its blinkers of arrogance were painfully blown off. It had doggedly ignored Indian experts' opinion which unfortunately wasn't given in strong enough language as they had felt scared of consequences of speaking honestly and forcefully.

For the central government fighting and winning elections was decidedly more important than saving lives of its citizens. With great difficulty and long wait the Hindutva fuelled political outfit governing at the centre had come to dominate the Indian political canvas and it didn't want to slow down its drive to continue and/or expand the same. It thought, though not expressing openly, that India wasn't short of human beings and a loss of few millions to the pandemic didn't make any difference. Experience had thought it that public memory was short, and the Hindutva enriched party had a large store of skilfully crafted slogans and/ or 'jumlas' to fool the public.

During its six years of governance, it had shamelessly broken bones of the key institutions designed to protect democracy and rule of law—namely judiciary, RBI and the Election Commission (EC) along with those of intellectuals who earlier spoke out to balance governance on democratic rails. It had gathered numerous tools and strategies to subdue people and institutions. EC had turned into an ally of the governing party since it willingly crafted election process to the advantage of ruling party. West Bengal election spread over to eight phases in March and April 2021 i.e., for full two months, was the greatest proof of the EC doing its masters' bidding. It provided BJP undue advantage of using/misusing government resources, all key ministers, and massive financial muscles to organise huge rallies and road shows and creating public impression that it had defeated the opposition even much before the voting process materialised. The suitably subdued media was its greatest ally. There wasn't any even-playing field available to the opposition. And uncontrolled use of coercive language and threats manipulated situation to benefit the party ruling at the centre.

The so-called Covid appropriate behaviour went into smoke and the smart Covid virus had a field day to infect and emerge as a huge wave. Poor public collected for huge rallies and road shows preferred the lure of cash and free food and drinks than to worrying about the pandemic. It suited the arrogance of ruling BJP. For it, rally grounds and huge stages weren't public place while a single individual in his personal car (without a mask) was viewed as have violated the sanctity of public place and such offenders were punished.

As per its Chief Minister, millions of people in Kumbh gatherings at Haridwar were said to be protected by the spirit of 'Ma Ganga'.

And massive gatherings in temples and festive celebrations like that of 'Holi' were immune to Covid danger as per utterances of Hindutva-stained politicians, priests, and sadhus.

For the misconceived thought line and expressions of the insensitive apparatus of governance the gullible Indian public paid dearly at hands of the Covid-19's vengeful avalanche in the 2nd quarter of 2021.

* * *

CORONA RECRUITED NEW WORRIERS TO ITS FIGHT AGAINST MANKIND

In a way the first phase of pandemic of the 21st century represented the battle of Kurukshetra where many kings and princes had joined on Duryodhana's side and Pandavas too got support of some who believed in power of righteousness. In similar fashion while mankind added some vaccines to help it, Covid (the modern day Duryodhana) recruited numerous variants or mutants to fight on its side. It had the celestial power to self-modify in a bid to survive and extend and intensify its fight. It was reported that the Wuhan virus had created over 2,700 variants by end of the 1st quarter of 2021. Of these the UK, Brazilian, South African and Indian variants were most vicious—and there were some locally minted double-variants. They acted fast, infecting, and killing indiscriminatingly, in addition to maiming those who survived. The aftereffects of Corona came to be known as 'Long-Covid'. The variants dodged vaccines in numerous ways, especially through rapid self-alterations. Even those who had taken both doses of the vaccines too got infected—and even newly born babies weren't spared. It seemed that Covid-19 through its variants gave a bloody nose to vaccines. At places like USA, Brazil, UK, South Africa, and India waves of infection were seen merging with each other and it was indeed difficult to see the same in form of second, third or fourth one. Especially, countries with inefficient and autocratic governance were hit the hardest. Hospitals were overwhelmed, running short of beds, ICUs, oxygen and ventilators—and dead bodies were seen piled-up in hospital corridors. Cremation ghats or grounds ran out of wood; electric ovens melted, and graveyards ran out of space. As per St. Hopkins University, officially reported deaths in the world had crossed three million mark by end of the 1st quarter of 2021. But as per author's assessment based on analysis of funeral and burial grounds' scenes, the actual loss of human lives during the period touched the level of 25-30 million—and by the time the dreaded pandemic decides to disappear or subside to a tolerable endemic in next 2-3 years the world would have lost more human lives than the early 20th century's Spanish flu's reported toll of 50 million. India's second wave (April through June 2021) had moved to its over 0.7 million villages killing a minimum of 25-30 people in each village; it had added up to loss of roughly over 40 million lives in just three months but the same weren't truthfully recorded to Covid account.

* * *

LARGE NUMBER OF DEAD BODIES FLOATED IN INDIA'S HOLY RIVERS

In May 2021, when the second wave of Covid-19 was yet to reach its peak, a large number of dead bodies were seen floating in Ganga and Yamuna which flow through the Hindutva ruled the high population density states of UP and Bihar. Villagers overwhelmed by the pandemic—and being short of wood and money needed for funerals just preferred to toss dead bodies into rivers. Ghastly scenes were captured by a few TV channels, not fully controlled by the Hindutva money bags—and a flood of criticism in media forced the two governments looking for cover. When pushed into corner, in face of lack of medicines and necessities like oxygen supply, 14 Chief Medical Officer (CMOs) in Unnao district, located just 40 km away from UP's capital Lucknow, had resigned en-mass.

In some cases, police were reported to have assisted villagers, through employment of their vans and JCV machines in tossing the dead bodies into river waters. Some of the bodies just fell on sand. Faced with a storm of criticism, some of the dead bodies were later pushed into hurriedly dug pits and then covered with loose sand. And dogs and wild animals were seen moving around such makeshift graves. National Human Rights Commission and the top court were seen demanding a thorough probe into the ghastly situation precipitated by the utter mismanagement of Covid pandemic by the two BJP ruled states. In earlier months both governments were seen fully gripped with elections unmindful of consequences.

* * *

BLACK FUNGUS EPIDEMIC EMERGED AS EXTENSION OF THE 2ND WAVE

Just when the 2nd Covid wave in India started to taper off black fungus infection in sinus cavities of patients recovering from the dreaded pandemic complicated the already serious situation. By the 3rd week of May 2021 over 9,000 such patients were officially reported in the country. Gujarat and Maharashtra were the two most seriously affected states. Patients were getting their eyes, jaws and brains affected; in several cases patients' eyes were removed. In some cases, patients lost their jaws and teeth. Terrible shortage of main medicine needed for treatment i.e., amphotericin B had created an unmanageable situation. And it came to light that mismanagement of Covid treatment with excessive use of steroids by inadequately trained and/or careless doctors, coupled with uncontrolled self-medication, especially in small towns and rural areas had led to uncontrolled surge of diabetics. High blood sugar situation lingering for long time allowed excessive fungus growth in patients recovering from Covid. The dreaded disease also affected children and a total lack of children specific ICUs complicated the situation. And some experts stated seeing the uncontrolled spread of the black fungus epidemic possibly as an early emergence of the 3rd wave.

* * *

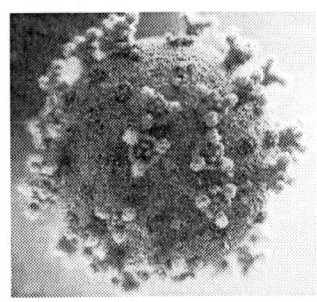

EPISODE 50

INDIA'S HIDDEN COVID-19 DEATHS

On 17 June 2021 "The Times of India" in its Delhi edition reported as under:

> "Centre refused nod to Delhi government to probe oxygen deaths." *An unhappy Delhi government reacted to say:*
>
> *"As a responsible government we want to offer compensation to the families of those who died and also investigate and confirm what led to these deaths."*

The government of India that controlled all important decisions of the NCT government apparently got scared of the outcome of such a probe. Such probes' outcome could have brought out the truth about the huge numbers of deaths hidden by various agencies of the Central Government. It could have had a chain reaction amongst the opposition ruled states. Such a situation could have overturned the apple cart of the Centre—and thus the cat could have jumped out of the bag of secrecy.

The truth about India's Covid-19 deaths presently remain hidden:

- In hospital records, small or big—and public and/or private ones scattered all over the country.

- In records of cremation and burial grounds of the thousands of small and big towns and over 7,00,000 villages.
- In records of mayors/ local governments of the small and big towns and those of numerous village panchayats; there wasn't any village, small and big, where 10, 15, 20, 30 or more deaths didn't occur during the second wave in April, May and June 2021.

The New York Times (as reported by The Times of India's Delhi edition dated May 27, 2021) based on surveys and opinion of distinguished experts reported that India's Covid-19 deaths were (a) twice of the officially announced figures as the most conservative estimate, (b) 16 lakh as the most likely case, and (c) 42 lakhs as the worst scenario.

And, as expected, the Indian government was critical of the NYT's opinion.

Hence, the truth about India's hidden deaths on account of Covid-19, in opinion of the author, shall never be known.

* * *

EPISODE 51

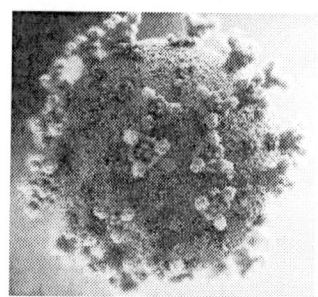

CERTAINTY OF THIRD WAVE IN INDIA

At end of June 2021 when the second wave subsided an analysis of circumstances led to believe that the arrival of the third wave in India in the 4th quarter of the year was almost certain because:

- India's large population allowed the virus to retain a large seed material which, on availability of suitable opportunities, would bounce back into a serious wave.
- Indian public isn't attuned to effective use of face masks because (a) the same aren't supplied free of cost and (b) the large sections of the population that fall below the poverty line find it difficult to spend money on this input for everyone in large families. And whatsoever masks are used by the massive majority of Indians are of poor quality, incapable of providing desired protection.
- India's living, travelling, and working conditions render observance of the 6 feet social distance entirely impossible. A large section of the population here lives in congested one room dwellings, each housing 5-6 individuals. Hence, if one catches the virus then eventually all of them are bound to contact the same.

- And India's social and medical safety net (by its very non-availability) does not allow poor families to take timely measures to treat or home quarantine the infected. Total non-availability of dependable medical facility in its over 7 lakh villages make the work of virus so very easy.
- India is unlikely to give up its super-spreading election events, religious gatherings and melas, and the traditional marriage sand festivals.
- India is also unlikely to vaccinate its two third or more population needed for effective herd immunity by the 4th quarter of the year.
- Corona is a great fighter. It hasn't yet given up its fight against humanity anywhere in the world. Then why should it walk out of India so early?
- Spanish flu had taken over 4 years to vacate its battlefield. Presently, the hugely congested world with wide-spread poverty and great air-connectivity allows the virus a much superior environment to fight a longer war.
- India's crowded markets and transports which offer super-spreading opportunities will not de-congest in a hurry.
- And the testing, tracing and home isolation practices shall not be able to rise to South Korean efficiency in a hurry.

Hence, India wouldn't be able put effective barricades in path of the dreaded virus. At end of June 2021 several experts, medical and/or otherwise, seemed to share and express similar thoughts regarding the inevitability of emergence of the third wave in the near future.

* * *

INDEX

Aam Admi Party (AAP), 172
Africa, 27, 51, 67, 88, 117, 146
Agra, 169
Ahmedabad, 143, 153, 169, 172
Air Travel, 76
Air-force One, 71
Arc de Triumph, 13
Arizona, 109, 131, 165
Artificial Intelligence (AI), 39, 63, 129
Arts, Artists, Galleries, 26
Asia, 27, 51, 67, 88, 117, 146
Assam, 174
Astha, 171, 175
Australia, 60, 107, 114, 123, 129
Austria, 6, 18, 63
Automation in business and industry, 101
Ayush ministry, 154

Bangladesh, 97
Belarus, 117
Belgium, 33, 65, 87, 109
Bengal Famine, 169
Bengaluru, 172
Bergamo, 2
Bhutan, 107, 142
Bihar, 144, 179
Black Lives Matter Agitation, 32, 132, 143, 165
Bolsonaro, Jair, Brazil's President, 30, 47, 67, 137

Brazil, 22, 29-30, 42, 45-46, 61-62, 68-69, 87, 103, 110, 127, 137, 143-44, 155, 178
British government, 143
British Mutant, 34

CAG, 173
California, 46, 109, 131
Canada, 35, 123
Catch 22 Situation, 134
CBI, 173
Central Asia, 108
Charles De-Gaulle, 13
Chennai, 135, 153, 172
Chicago, 122
China, 2-4, 9, 12, 20, 26, 52-53, 59, 61, 72, 103, 107, 113-14, 118, 125-29, 166
Chinese Virus, 53, 157, 162, 164
Consumer goods, 24
Coronavirus, 99, 103, 111, 132, 158
    Origin, 157
Coronil, 154
Co-Vaccine, 127
Covid-19, 7, 9, 15, 17-18, 20-26, 31, 34, 36, 38, 41, 43-46, 48-51, 54, 56, 58-59, 63, 65-67, 73, 75-76, 80, 95, 100-01, 105-06, 108-10, 121-26, 129-30, 133, 136-38, 140, 142, 144, 146-47, 150, 152, 154-56, 158, 163, 170, 176, 179, 181

Dangerous Digital Divide, 50

Dark Winter, 56-57, 70, 120
Delhi, 135, 143, 153, 169, 172
Denmark, 6, 63
Disaster Management Act, 44
Distance Education, 25
Dr Anthony Fauci, 31, 68, 73, 132, 160
Dr Gopinath, IMF, 160
Dr R. Bright, 31, 56-57
Dr Rick Bright, 55
Dr. Harsh Vardhan, India's Health Minister, 173
Dragon's conspiracy, 113

Economy, 100
Education, 102
Election Commission (EC), 176
Europe, 8, 11, 18, 22, 27, 61, 63, 66, 69, 81, 109, 126, 132-33, 145, 160
European Union (EU), 8, 10, 103, 115 Administration, 6

FB, 75
Finland, 63
Florida, 109, 131, 165
France, 7, 13, 18, 36, 61, 63-64, 70, 87, 95, 109, 115, 139, 141
Frankfurt, 122
French Economy, 13

G-20, 25
G-7, 25
Games arenas, 26
Germany, 6-7, 18, 33-34, 61, 63-65, 87, 109, 126, 131, 133, 139
Ghaziabad, 169
Globalisation, 93, 99-100
Government of India (GOI), 37-38, 153-54
Greece, 34, 64
Gujarat, 145, 180
Gurugram, 169, 172

Health Infrastructure, 101
Hong Kong, 59, 117

Hospitality Industry, 92
Human
  Beings, 106
  Capital, 102
  Societies, 92, 133
Humanity, Cultural Capital, 101
Hydroxy Chloroquine (HCQ), 111, 158

ICMR, 114, 127
ICUs, 13, 16, 28, 44, 61, 71, 172, 175, 178, 180
IMF, 118, 148
India, 29, 37, 42, 46, 61, 69-71, 87-88, 97, 103, 117, 126-27, 135-37, 143, 146, 153, 166, 178, 184
  Second Wave, 112
Indian Festival, 26
Indian Lockouts, 80
Indian Navy ships, 81
Indian Railways, 145
International Co-operation, 25
International Court of Justice (ICJ), 53
Iran, 1-2, 5, 30, 61, 153, 162
Israel, 132
Italy, 1-2, 4-5, 8, 12, 21, 33, 36, 61, 64, 95, 109, 115, 139, 141, 162-63

Jaipur, 172
Japan, 1, 5, 88, 107, 114, 126, 161-62
Johnson, Boris, 15-16, 97, 140, 143
Jugad, 16

Kerala, 174
Kumbh Mela, 171
Kurukshetra, 153

Latin America, 51, 117
Little Flu, 30, 45, 67
Lockdowns, 28, 82-83, 85, 95-97, 106-07, 138, 150
  Frustrate People, 85
Lombardy, 4
London, 122

INDEX

Long Covid, 19, 178
LORR, 27-29, 151
Lucknow, 169, 172

Macron, French President, 54
Madrid, 122
Maharashtra, 180
Malaysia, 1, 5, 162
Manufacturing Industry, 24
Mental Health Situation, 102
Mexico, 69
Middle East, 81
Migrant Workers, 84
   Movement, 24
Milan's City Square, 6
Milano, 33, 122
Mismanagement, 45, 142
Moderna, 128
Modi, Narendra, Indian Prime Minister, 71, 168
Modi Government, 42
Morrison, Scott, Australian Prime Minister, 3
Moscow, 20, 142
Multi-organ Inflammation, 48
Mumbai, 135, 143, 153, 172

National Capital Region (NCR), 29
National Human Rights Commission, 179
NDA Government, 80, 84
Netherlands, 6, 18, 65
New Central Vista, 172
New Poverty, 7
New South Wales, 130
New York, 73, 103, 122, 140, 143, 163-64
New York Times, 182
New Zealand, 59-60, 88, 107, 123, 129, 139, 142
NHS, 16
Nigeria, 97
North America, 67
Northern Italy, 2

OPEC, 25
Oxford-Astra-Zeneca, 128
Oxygen, 178

Pakistan, 1, 5, 61, 88-89, 153
Paris, 122
Patna, 169, 172
People co-operated, 43
Peru, 62, 144
Pfizer Vaccine, 18
Pharma Industry, 102
Philippines, 30
Planning Commission of India, 173
Portugal, 109
Post-Corona Societies, 118
post-Covid-19, 101, 159
post-Lockdown 2.0, 79
PPEs, 2, 10, 13, 16, 21-23, 28, 31, 39, 44, 59-61, 71-72, 89, 108, 111, 114, 126, 140, 145-46, 155, 161, 163
pre-Covid-19, 100-01
   Global Operations, 24
President Putin, 20-22
President Trump, 29, 31, 53, 57, 70-72, 74-75, 96-97, 109, 111, 119-20, 127, 137, 140, 148, 155, 161-62
Puducherry, 174

RBI, 173, 176
Religious gatherings, 25
Respiratory Failure, 154
Russia, 20-21, 30, 70, 87, 117, 128, 142-44, 166

Saudi Arabia, 108
Saviour, 170
Second Wave, 33
Self-reliance, 24
Singapore, 1, 5, 60, 88, 107, 123, 130, 161-62
Social Capital, Charities and Compassion, 101

South Africa, 61, 127, 178
South America, 67, 88-89, 146
South Asia, 107
South Korea, 1, 5, 59-60, 88, 107, 123, 139, 161-62
Southern Europe, 27, 141
Spain, 1, 2, 5-7, 9-11, 18, 33, 36, 61, 64-65, 70, 87, 95-96, 109, 115, 132-33, 139, 141, 162-63
Spain's bull fighting festivities, 9
Spanish Flu, 169, 184
Sports, 101
Sputnik-V, 22, 129
Sri Lanka, 59, 107
St. Hopkins University, 178
St. Peters' Square, Rome, 6, 39
Stay Alert, 97
Struggling oil prices, 94
Super-spreader, 119
Surat, 169, 172
Sweden, 63, 86, 95

Taiwan, 5, 59, 88, 114, 123, 139, 142, 161-62
Tamil Nadu, 174
Teaching Methods, 25
Texas, 109, 131, 165
The Times of India, 181-82
Tiny Flu, 47
Tourism, 77, 92
Trump Administration, 68
Trump's 'America First', 93
Trump's Mishandling, 137
Turkey, 30, 62, 153
Twitter, 75

UK Government, 18

UN Operations, 25
UN-based Organisations, 93
Unemployment, 4, 92
United Kingdom (UK), 7, 10, 15, 17-18, 27, 34, 36, 60-61, 64-66, 69-70, 95, 109, 126, 128, 131, 133, 140, 142-43, 166-67, 178
UNO, 118
UP, 144, 179
US/USA, 2-3, 6, 22, 26-27, 29-30, 36, 42, 45, 56, 60-61, 68-69, 87, 89, 95, 103, 109, 113, 118, 122, 126, 131, 137, 144, 150, 152, 155, 163, 166-67, 178
    Administration, 162
    Media, 73

Varanasi, 169
Ventilators, 13, 31, 61, 108, 126, 178
Victoria, 130
Vietnam, 59-60, 123, 139, 161
Vishva Guru, 38, 42, 170, 175

West, 60
West Bengal, 174
    Election, 176
Whistle-blower, 55
White House, 35
Workers, Jobless and Homeless, 82
World Food Output, 101
World Health Organization (WHO), 1-2, 26, 31, 41, 52-53, 58, 69, 74, 115, 118, 126, 152-53, 157, 161-62, 166-67, 171
WTO, 72
Wuhan, 5, 12, 20, 27, 30-31, 52, 59, 103, 125, 129, 138, 141, 158

Xi Jinping, 30